AF826051

Blair Ashby

Talking Man to Man

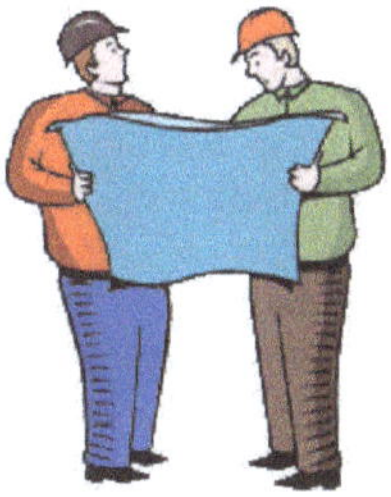

About facing your own stuff, dealing with pain, loss, and depression then getting on with your life

Blair Ashby **Talking Man to Man**

About facing your own stuff,
dealing with pain, loss, and depression
then getting on with your life

Published by
E&R Productions
Denver, Colorado

Text, graphics, and cover art copyright 2010-2013 by Blair Ashby.
All rights reserved.

ISBN: 978-0-9847373-7-6
1. Health & Fitness, 2. Self Help, 3. Body Mind & Spirit, 4. Author, 5. Title

Library of Congress Catalog-in-Publication data available upon request from service@eddlesenrowe.com.

All rights reserved
Printed in the United States of America
E&R Productions is a division of Eddlesen & Rowe, LLC

No part of this publication can be reproduced, stored in any retrieval systems, or transmitted in any form or by any means, electronic, mechanical, photocopying, recording, scanning, or otherwise, except as permitted under Section 107 or 108 of the 1976 United States Copyright Act, without prior written permission of the author.

Trademarks: Talking Man to Man logos are trademarks of the author. All other trademarks referred to herein are trademarks of Eddlesen & Rowe, LLC or its affiliates.

Limit of Liability/Disclaimer of Warranty: The advice and strategies contained herein may not be suitable for your situation. You should consult with a professional or a medical practitioner when appropriate. The author and publisher of this book specifically disclaim any implied warranties of merchantability or fitness for a particular purpose of the contents of this book. No warranty may be created or extended by sales representatives or written sales materials. Neither the publisher nor the author shall be liable for any loss of profit or any other personal or commercial damages, including but not limited to special, incidental, consequential, or other damages.

10 9 8 7 6 5 4 3 2 1

This book is dedicated to my Dad, Maurice,
for teaching me about being a man and
to my daughter, Kari, for teaching me it's not
always about manliness.

Talking Man to Man

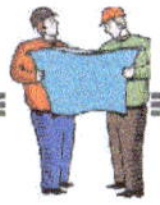

Tools In The Toolbox

(All the Tools in one place)

TOOL #1 – NOT THIS!

If you're reading this book, you, or someone you know, is probably experiencing some kind of darkness. You're probably feeling anger, grief, cheated, betrayed, lost, depressed, disconnected, or some other type of negative emotion.
If you want to move out of this darkness, one of the first steps you can take is to recognize NOT THIS!

"Not this" simply means you don't want to be here and won't accept being stuck here! Realizing you don't have to stay in this darkness is vital! You can move out of the dark into a full and happy life!

You're at a crossroads. You have a decision to make about your future life. Your choices are: do you want relief or do you want happiness? Most men choose relief. It's easier and faster – for a while. A few men, however, want more. They want happiness – even though it's harder work and usually takes longer to achieve.

"Not This!" is your first step. Choosing long term happiness or short term relief is your second step. Choose wisely. Courage is needed no matter what you decide.

For more info, go to ***Keep Your Fingers On The Wall***, page 1.

TOOL #2 – FEEL THE BURN, BUT YOU ARE NOT THE BURN

Once you can see your darkness as something you feel, and you can accept your darkness as a feeling you are having and not a definition of who you are, you can start to be in it and overcome it.

Let me explain. When you smash your thumb with a hammer, you feel pain! You are not the pain!

Darkness is the same way, although we men like to think differently. We FEEL depressed, we aren't depressed. We FEEL anger, we are not angry. We FEEL betrayed, we are not betrayed. Emotions are a sensation in our bodies. They are not us. We only feel them.

By learning to separate yourself from the emotions you feel, you start to build an identity for yourself based on WHO you are, not what you are. Only then can you start to find your way out of the darkness you FEEL.

For more info go to ***Feel The Burn…You Are Not What You Feel***, page 9.

TOOL #3 – SHUT UP! AND LISTEN TO YOURSELF!

How many sounds can you hear right now? The TV, the game on the radio, the kids playing, the office humming? If you're out to eat, the TV in the bar is going and in the dining area music is going. We live in a noisy world!

Ironically, most of that noise is self induced to hide behind. We hate to be in silence. Why is that? If you're like most men, it's because noise drowns out the running commentary in your mind. So we turn on the saw, start the mower, crank the MP3 . . .

Now, try concentrating on something. Notice how quiet it gets in your mind when you focus. How much more space does your brain have to think in with all that quietness? Have you ever noticed that a problem's solution frequently comes when you're not thinking about the problem?

Pick an activity, sport, or hobby and focus on it. Spend some time concentrating only on it. Give your brain space to chew through the noise in your life and find the dreams hidden below the racket. When it's ready, your mind will bring the reasons for your darkness up to the conscious mind for you to work through to happiness.

For more info go to ***Shut Up! And Listen To Yourself***, page 19.

TOOL#4 – EPIPHANIES TAKE TIME

Here's some good news: If you keep searching inside for the reasons you feel this darkness, you will find the answers and then you can fix the problems. Here's some news that isn't so fun: This process can take time. If this was easy, you would have found the solution long ago and never needed to subject yourself to this darkness to begin with.

Unfortunately, we live in a self-created, noisy world to hide from our inner commentary telling us we missed a goal somewhere. Thus, it takes time to hear through all that noise, to the still small voice which is telling you what you need to do to get your life back on the right track.

Have patience with yourself. Have patience with the process. Yes, I realize that sucks! Answers NOW are so much easier. However, quick answers rarely last a lifetime. The tools of listening to yourself and having patience with the process does last a lifetime. Epiphanies take time. The better life and happiness you'll enjoy because of it will be worth it.

For more info go to ***Epiphanies Take Time***, page 29.

TOOL #5 – YOU GOTTA GROW ON

Chances are, your way of doing things are what brought you to this dark place in your life to begin with. It certainly was for me. I kept making small "quick and easy" sacrifices until one day my dreams for my life said "HEY! WHAT ABOUT ME?"

At that point, I started down the path that led me to discover I had made these sacrifices all the way to failure. I had a choice to make. Do I keep doing what I've done to more failure? Or, do I examine what I did wrong, and let go of my old ways (which didn't work) to make room for new models of success?

Believe it or not, it was hard to let go of the old programs. But I had to move beyond them if I was going to be happy again.

You have to make this same decision. Make the choice to leave behind the old methods which don't work any more and move into new models which leave you space to live a full and happy life.

For more info go to ***You Gotta Grow On***, page 37.

TOOL #6 – JUST DO SOMETHING!

As I was growing up, when I got stuck on a project, my dad used to say to me, "Just do something. Because even if it's wrong, you'll learn from the mistakes and that'll get you closer to right."

He was right. When you're stuck in darkness, force yourself to move in the direction where you think your dreams are. There's a high probability you'll not get it right the first time, but you will force yourself to learn. From those efforts, you will gain things that bring you closer to your goals and your happiness.

For a story about this, go to ***Just Do Something***, page 45.

TOOL #7 – DEAL WITH YOUR STUFF!

What is your stuff? Let me explain. When I was in depression, I'd complain about all the people, situations, and wrong outcomes making my life unbearable. I'd have an excuse for every miserable thing that was happening to me. Then, one day, a client of mine told me that the hardest thing he had to learn during his mid-life crisis was "What's my stuff?"

We men have a tendency to put responsibility for our lives on somebody or something else. Life happens to us. Then, when it happens "wrong" we complain because we think we're the victim.

Instead, we should ask ourselves what's our part in these situations. We can't control other variables. However, we can control us. Our actions, our responses, our expectations. That's our stuff!

When we acknowledge our place in our life, we take on the ability to control our feelings about the things we experience. So, what's your stuff?

- Own your responsibility.
- Own your attachments to events, people, places and/or outcomes.
- Own your expectations!
- Own your life and happiness!

For more info go to ***Deal With Your Stuff***, page 51.

TOOL #8 – WHAT DO YOU REALLY, REALLY, REALLY WANT?

Here's a simple fact: if you don't know what you want, you can't go for it. In the big scheme of your life, what do you really, really, really want?

Big TVs, boats, and fast cars don't fall into this question. They're fairly shallow endeavors. Compared to things like your life, your family and relationships, and your legacy, a motorcycle just doesn't belong in the equation.

However, this question is also about boundaries. Life has restrictions and those restrictions are probably a big part of the darkness you're feeling now. If you don't know what you want, you will still end up somewhere in life but with boundaries you didn't choose consciously.

What do you really, really, really want? Choose wisely. Choose courageously. Choose your dreams and choose your boundaries. Choose to live the life you want while being conscious of the restrictions which come with your choice.

For more info go to ***What Do You Really, Really, Really Want?***, page 61.

TOOL# 9 – WINNING BY YIELDING

Whether big or small, part of what you really, really, really want is related to the sacrifices you need to make to accomplish that goal. For instance, if your goal is to get home safe and relaxed at the end of the day, does it further your goal to race through traffic, risking your life and other's for a ten second gain . . . not to mention the added stress of being the wack-job on the road.

My friend, Scott, calls this *Winning by Yielding*. If you know your important goals, it's much easier to sacrifice the small, unimportant distractions to achieve your larger dreams.

For more info read ***Winning by Yielding***, page 69.

TOOL #10 – KEEP ON FALLING

Imagine you've fallen into a mighty rushing river, found a big boulder, and you're clinging to it against the onslaught of the water. You hold desperately to that rock fearing the consequences of letting go and being carried away by the flow.

Now imagine trusting your swimming abilities, and instead of clinging to the rock, you push yourself off from it into the smoothest part of the river. As you traverse the distance, look up and see the canyon, watch the scenery, enjoy the trip. When an obstacle appears in front of you, use it as guidance and an opportunity.

Life is constantly flowing. You can fight it, but you're still in it. Shouldn't you try to experience all that life can bring you. If you cling to some perceived security, you will be bashed and battered and constantly reacting to life's happenings.

If you let go into the flow of life, you will be able to respond proactively to the things life brings to you. You will have the awareness to know your goals and the steps you need to take to accomplish them. You will have the freedom to live your life to it's fullest – choosing your path, your feelings, your happiness.

For more information go to ***Never Stop Falling***, page 81.

Blair Ashby

Talking Man to Man

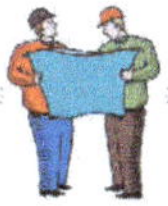

Table of Contents

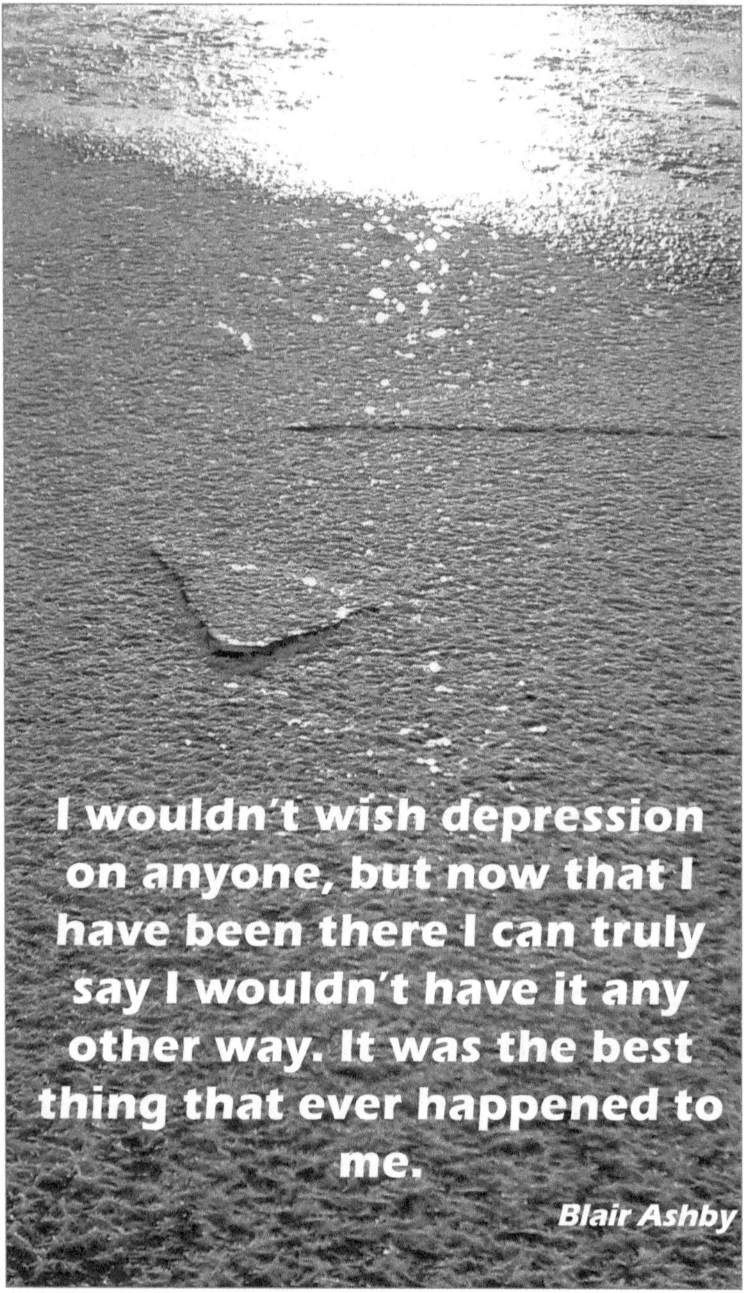
I wouldn't wish depression on anyone, but now that I have been there I can truly say I wouldn't have it any other way. It was the best thing that ever happened to me.
Blair Ashby

Ice Wedge by Blair Ashby

Foreword
by Fred Berns

That *Talking Man to Man* has a profound impact on me comes as no surprise.

Blair Ashby has had that impact on me for years.

He has been a source of inspiration and light, and a voice of reason dating back to the time, years ago, when I hired him to help me create and produce audio products for my speaking and training business.

I was impressed from the outset, not only by his technical capabilities, but by his dedication and commitment to service. His was more than "service with a smile." It was a passion for excellence and a sincere interest in my success.

Gradually, as we continued to work together, conversations transcended the project at hand. We began discussing larger issues – such as the challenges of running a business and of work and personal relationships.

The conversations were never long, due to the deadlines and responsibilities that we both faced as business owners. But I always found the brief discussions meaningful and memorable. So much so, that I looked forward to each opportunity to get together with Blair to share our lives in general, and personal issues in particular.

I began to view Blair as a sounding board and as an advisor on the good, bad, and ugly of relationships in my role of husband, father, and friend to my friends. That, in itself, is significant considering how rare it is for guys to open up to one another about their personal lives.

Connecting with Blair helped fill the void and gave me the opportunity, once again, to discuss weighty issues on a man-to-man level – weighty issues like relationships with my wife, son, and elderly parents, pressures to succeed financially, etc.

What impresses me about Blair is his ability to focus on the root cause of a problem and respond to that problem with clarity and insights. I have benefited time and time again from those insights and from the way he has personalized and customized his wisdom to my situation.

Blair has a flair – for hearing as well as listening and for coming up with simple answers to complicated questions. As a professional communicator, I know the importance of economizing on words and speaking succinctly. Blair does, too.

Not long ago, I shared with Blair one of life's most common, yet complicated challenges: a communication breakdown. I mentioned to him how verbal interaction between my wife and I wasn't as good as it could be, and should be.

Blair did what he does so well: he helped me put the problem in perspective and reminded me of the importance of tolerance, understanding, and taking responsibility for my thoughts, actions, and relationships.

He convince me to confront the verbal breakdown head-on (rather than just accept it, as I had done) and take steps to restore lines of communication. He told me to come to terms with, and deal with, my "shit," before condemning my wife for hers.

It worked like a charm. Following my "heart to heart" talk with my wife, our level of verbal give-and-take improved quickly and substantially.

The experience convinced me that other men could benefit a great deal from Blair's advice. I figured if he could guide me through my darkness, he could bring about similar results with other men. Which is what led me to suggest to Blair, one afternoon while we were drinking beer, that he write a book.

Who better than an enlightened guy to write a book on how guys can become more enlightened? Who better to advise men on how to confront and move beyond their personal darkness than a man who had been there, done that?

I am honored and overjoyed that Blair took my advice and responded proactively to the encouragement of others to share his wisdom with a wider audience.

"I can't give you answers. Nobody can," Blair points out early in *Talking Man to Man*. "The only thing I can give you are signposts that will point you in the right direction."

Blair has given me a whole lot of signposts in recent years. I am sure that through this powerful book, he will supply you with a great many signposts as well.

Fred Berns is a branding coach, copywriter, and speaker who helps companies dramatically differentiate themselves and master their marketplace. He offers coaching and speaking programs, and marketing and branding campaigns. Fred can be reached at www.whatsyouronly.com

"Tell them what only you do and they will buy only from you."

Introduction

by Alan J. Parisse MBA, CSP, CPAE

Real men don't ask for directions. My dad never did. He knew where he was going and would figure out how to get there. Or at least that's how it seemed to me. So, like most men I know, I developed a "go it alone" mentality. Oh, I had a couple of mentors and some great friends, but when the chips were down, I kept it close to the vest.

Support groups? Not for real men. Religious institutions? I tried a few. The people were great, but it didn't do the trick. Self-help books? Good ideas, yet they seemed to be talking to someone else.

This book is different. As the title says, it is *Talking Man to Man* – and it is high time someone did. It's kind of two books in one.

One is the story of a real man's decline into darkness and his journey back out to the light. It is about how he hit the skids, tried to go it alone and found he couldn't do it. Fortunately for him and for everyone who reads this book, he sank low enough to finally admit he had a problem. Then, and only then, he found the help he needed to rise from the smoldering ashes of his former life and find a new and better one.

The second book is a road map for the rest of us to either avoid the trip down or to catch ourselves a lot sooner should we fall.

Blair Ashby is the perfect person to have written this book. He is not a spiritual leader, but he has professionally recorded some of the finest and taken their words to heart. He is not a shrink, but he has been to one whom he credits with helping him break out of his funk and find meaning in his life.

Instead, Blair is a real guy who has "been there – done that" and come out the other end to live the life he wanted.

Without doubt, this book is a must read for any man who finds himself stressed by financial or personal problems or diminished by the feeling that his life dreams are fading out of reach.

Frankly, however, it may be almost as important for men whose lives are just fine to read this book and keep it on the shelf. That way, if – or more likely when – the cycles of life catch up with them, they will be ready.

The book is designed to be read the way most men read books – a few punchy pages at a time. It is chock full of action ideas to help us let go of the past and start moving to our new future. In Blair's words, to what we "really, really, really want."

By the way, my Dad never asked for directions, but I use

my GPS. I'll bet you do also. So think of this book as a GPS for your life.

Alan J. Parisse MBA, CSP, CPAE
"One of the Top 21 Speakers for the 21st Century"
Successful Meetings Magazine

The Parisse Group, Inc.
www.parisse.com

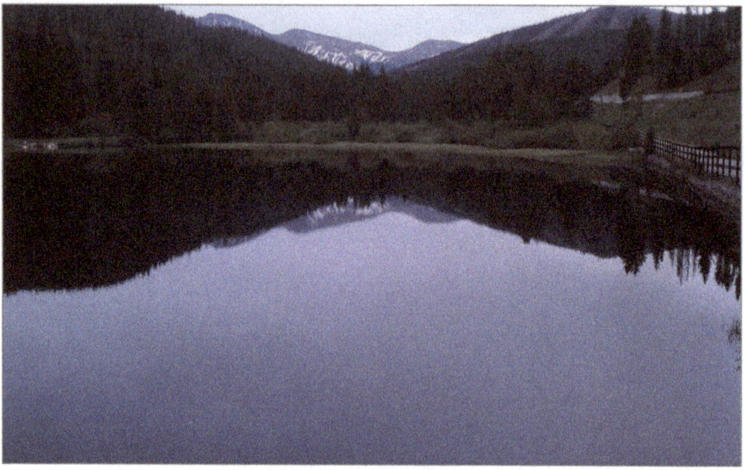

Imagine Your Perfect Life...

Winter Park Lake Reflection by Blair Ashby

Picture Your Life At Its Best

I guess most men would say:

- My wife is hot and my sex life is to die for.
- My kids are the best athletes and/or, the smartest kids in school.
- I drive the hottest car.
- I have a great retirement fund built up.
- I own the house they show on television.
- I take five weeks of vacation fishing each year.
- I make enough to buy anything I want.
- My life is only going to get better.
- I'm headed for the corner office where I'll golf four times a week and the rest of the time I'll be in the office acting like I'm actually doing something and getting paid for it.
- My kids will go to the best universities on full ride scholarships.

Nice huh?

But let's face it. Life's not always that way. Life frequently sucks.

And those dreams you had when you were growing up,

when you were in high school, when you were in college . . . little by little, you begin to sacrifice those dreams. You're always doing it for something better, of course – your wife, your marriage, your kids. You work a bit more so you can make a bit more money to get a better house, a better car, a better life for your family, whatever.

Invariably, you end up making thousands of little sacrifices. These sacrifices steal your dreams away from you until one day, your life is a shell of what you wanted it to be.

Okay, so you probably have a good life. You probably make enough money to do mostly what you want. You get your vacation time. Your boss is happy. Your wife is beautiful. Your kids are doing okay . . . maybe.

You're not going to the corner office and chances are when you come home at the end of the day, you walk in, you drop your briefcase, you throw your jacket on the chair and you say, "Hi, I'm home. What's for dinner?" Then you go plop down in front of that stupid television, turn it on, and turn your brain off for the next six hours until you go to bed. And the next morning, you start the drudgery again.

You are disappointed, maybe even a little angry about how things turned out. Okay, maybe a lot angry. You feel helpless. Out of control. Depressed. Victimized. Cheated. Betrayed. In short, you are suffering in some way or another.

You are not alone.

I had a millionaire stand in my studio the other day and tell me about a 12 year court case he was in against his brother – over money.

I had a client walk into my studio, an angry broken man. When I asked him what was up, he told me he was sick to death of everything his wife did wrong. The next morning he was going to sit her down and let her know how wrong she was.

The happiest man I know sat down in front of me not long ago and started to cry because his wife had a stroke and the woman he married doesn't exist anymore.

I stopped to see some long-time neighbors. The husband wasn't home at the time, but I talked to the wife for a few minutes. She told me that six months previously her husband had been jumped in a gas station by two guys. One of them came up behind my neighbor and smashed his head down into the car so hard it knocked him out as the other thief rifled through my friend's wallet. The thief got $60. Now my neighbor has permanent brain damage and has post-it notes everywhere to try to remind him to do even the most basic tasks.

I watched my friends get divorced, declare bankruptcy, lose their houses, lose their kids, lose their jobs, lose their loved ones, lose their dreams.

I have been all those men. And I expect you have too.

Now you look at me and say, "Geez, thanks, Blair. Where can I find a brick to throw at you for all that cheery stuff?" But I know, and you know, that life is frequently not about cheery stuff.

So what happened?

What happened to the fun? What happened to going off for a fun weekend in Vegas or New York? What happened to the house they do television shows about? That amazing house that never needs painting and never needs maintenance? The car that never breaks? The job that's always fulfilling? What happened?

We just came through what historians say was "the great recession," and you may be angry because you lost your job. You may be pissed off because you lost your house or your car. You may be sad because you lost your wife. You may be frustrated with your kids. You may be jaded because you just got back from serving your country in a war zone and no one seems to care about your missing arm or leg or mind or soul.

And what do you do now?

While you are thinking about that, let me tell you my story.

2008 was the best year I ever had financially. So I decided

to take the first two weeks of 2009 off to improve my guitar skills. On January 3rd, I walked into my studio and I noticed a gray mist around everything. I didn't think much of it except maybe my contacts were dirty. It certainly wasn't dark outside. I seem to remember it was a sunny day.

On January 4, the mist was a little darker. a little grayer. A little thicker. And on January 5, it was worse again.

On January 6, when I came home from the studio, my wife asked me, "How was your day?" For the first time I answered," It was a dark day. I'm in a dark place, but I'll be okay in a day of two."

On the 7th and 8th, the days turned to charcoal. The mist became a thick fog. And on January 9th I descended into the valley of the shadow of death. I descended into the dark night of the soul. The darkest period of my life.

In the middle of March 2009, the national recession had been going full bore, and I was three months into my own personal recession. In 2008, I had one client who spent $42,000 with me. In 2009, that same client spent $200. That is a recession!

Then one day, all of a sudden, the cloud lifted off of me. I had a brief moment of clarity when I could see myself. I recognized what was happening.

I was standing in the kitchen leaning against the stove

while my wife was fixing dinner. I was pissing and moaning about how dark it was and how unhappy and miserable I was. She told me that I had to get help and I told her I didn't need help. I could make it on my own.

Suddenly, I stopped and said, "Sheri." She turned to look at me. I went over and took her face in my hands and I said, "Listen to me fast. If I don't get better in two weeks, you have to get help for me because I'm going to a very bad place."

What I hadn't told her that day in March was that I had taken out a half million dollar life insurance policy and picked a mountain to drive off. For some reason, in that brief, clear moment, I realized what I was going to do.

Two weeks later, the first of many extraordinary events happened. And these events would keep happening every two weeks for the next several months.

A visit by my friend, Jim, was the first. He said, "What you don't know about me, Blair, is that in my former life I was a therapist." And, "Wow, Blair, you're in depression."

I stared at him. At that moment, I recognized the truth in his words. He went on by saying, "I can tell you two things. This won't mean anything to you now, but you're going to get better. The other is, don't be afraid to be where you're at and feel. Learn from it."

I started to bawl when he said that.

The last thing I wanted to do was feel this way or learn from it.

Yet at that moment, I remembered a book I'd read many years earlier which said if you put your hand on the wall of a maze and you start walking, even in pitch blackness you'll always find your way out of the maze.

After my conversation with Jim, a few other key people walked into my life. These people – and except for once, it was always men – gave me the tools to start moving forward again.

Because the tools given to me gave me some direction out of my darkness, I have written this book to give these tools to you.

If you're reading this, it's because in some aspect of your life, you too are experiencing this darkness.

Maybe you are the man who lost his job, his income, his retirement. Maybe you are the man whose wife has left him. Maybe you are the man whose kids are failing school. Maybe you are the man who came back from the service with physical and mental scars so deep it seems like they will never heal.

Now, I'm not going to tell you that this will be easy. I'm not going to tell you you'll get better right away. And I'm not going to try to give you answers.

When people did that to me, I wanted to smack them with a 2x4 alongside their heads and watch their eyeballs pop out. I hated it when well-meaning people would look at me and say:

"It will be okay in the end."
"This too shall pass."
"Just change the way you're thinking."
"Just change your attitude."

What did they know about this? What did they know about what I was going through? What did they know about me?

I hated the power of positive thinking and all that crap. And why the hell is it called a "secret" if everyone knows it? Are you serious. I'm in the middle of a depression here, and they think I'm just going to go off and think happy balloon thoughts and that'll make it all better?

When you are in the middle of suffering, the last thing you want to hear is people saying stupid platitudes!

Because it's not going to be okay. When you're in the middle of that kind of hell, positive thinking means nothing to you. You don't know where the end is. And if I said I did, you would say, "Go away Blair, you don't know anything."

The fact of the matter is, the only way you're going to get out of your suffering is if you go through it. And the only way you're going to do that is if you stop looking for answers in the light.

Here is one of my favorite stories.

One night, a man saw his neighbor looking for something

under the streetlight. “What are you looking for?” the man asked.

“My keys,” the other replied. Being a good neighbor the man decided to help with the search.

After a time of futile searching the man, who was anxious to get home, asked, “Are you sure this is where you lost your keys?”

“Oh no,” replied the neighbor, “I lost them over there near the hedge.”

The man was stunned. “Then why are you looking for your keys here?” he demanded.

“Because the light is better over here,” his neighbor answered.

This is an ancient story. One that has been told many times in many different ways. I had heard it before, but in the past, I always thought the man looking for his keys was an imbecile.

Suddenly, I got it. I thought, “So why the hell are you looking in the light, Blair? Maybe because it’s easier?”

The answer isn’t in the light. You need to look in your darkness, in your suffering.

Here’s the real deal. When you’re lost in the dark, your

important truths aren't found in the light. You have to be in your darkness and look blindly in that dark to find your answers which will then help you to escape your hell.

The only answers you will find are inside you and the only way you'll find them is by yourself.

One of my favorite quotes is from Dante. "Midway through my life, I came into a dark wood and the path was wholly lost."

That was me, lost in the darkness. And that is probably you, too.

During those dark days, my friend Warren told me, "Blair, at this point in your life you want the Star Trek transporter to transport you into the future when this is all over. But you can't go there because that transporter doesn't exist."

He was right. I wanted that transporter. I wanted relief. I didn't want to suffer. I didn't want to hurt. I didn't want to constantly fear for my stupid credit rating or my failing marriage or whether I was going to get the next bill paid or not.

I wanted hints that told me it was going to be okay. For me, the hints had to be something very tangible, very believable and, eventually, I found my clues.

In my case, the hints came in the form of coins – hundreds and hundreds of coins. I found them everywhere, in the most extraordinary times and places. Every time I found a coin, I picked it up, and for a brief second the fog would clear and I would believe that things would be okay. God's change, I called them.

Your clues will probably be different. However, when you find it, take it as positive re-enforcement that you're going to make it.

I also searched through everything for help: poets and philosophers, the great authors, the writings of inspirational and spiritual teachers, and the lectures of well known speakers.

I wanted someone to give me a set of tools that I could use – all in one place.

This is the book I wished someone had written for me.

I can't give you answers, though. Nobody can. The only thing I can give you are signposts that point you in the right direction. I can give you hints to paths that you can choose to walk.

The tools in this book are just reflectors in the storm to guide you toward the end of the journey – toward happiness.

When you're driving through an amazing storm, and you have to get from point A to point B, and you can't see three feet in front of your windshield, the reflector poles on the side of the road are there. Every tenth of a mile.

No matter how fast or how slow you're going, for a brief instant, when you're passing one, you know you're on the right path. You know, for a moment, it is going to be okay.

Then it's gone and you're in darkness again, but only until the next one, a 10th of a mile later. And then you pass the next one, and the next one, and the next one. You realize you're going to make it, that you can make it safely home.

Three months ago, I sat in a restaurant having lunch with my dad. He looked at me and said, "You know, Blair, I think you're happier now than you have been in the past ten years."

And he's right.

And that's what I want for you, the reader of this book. That when you get through your darkness (hopefully using some of the tools in this book) you can look back and say, "I'm moving forward with my life and my dreams. I'm happier than I've ever been before."

Blair Ashby

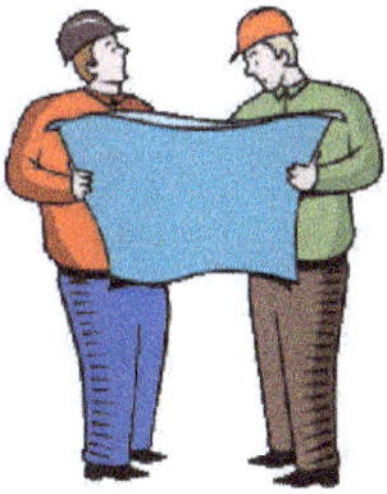

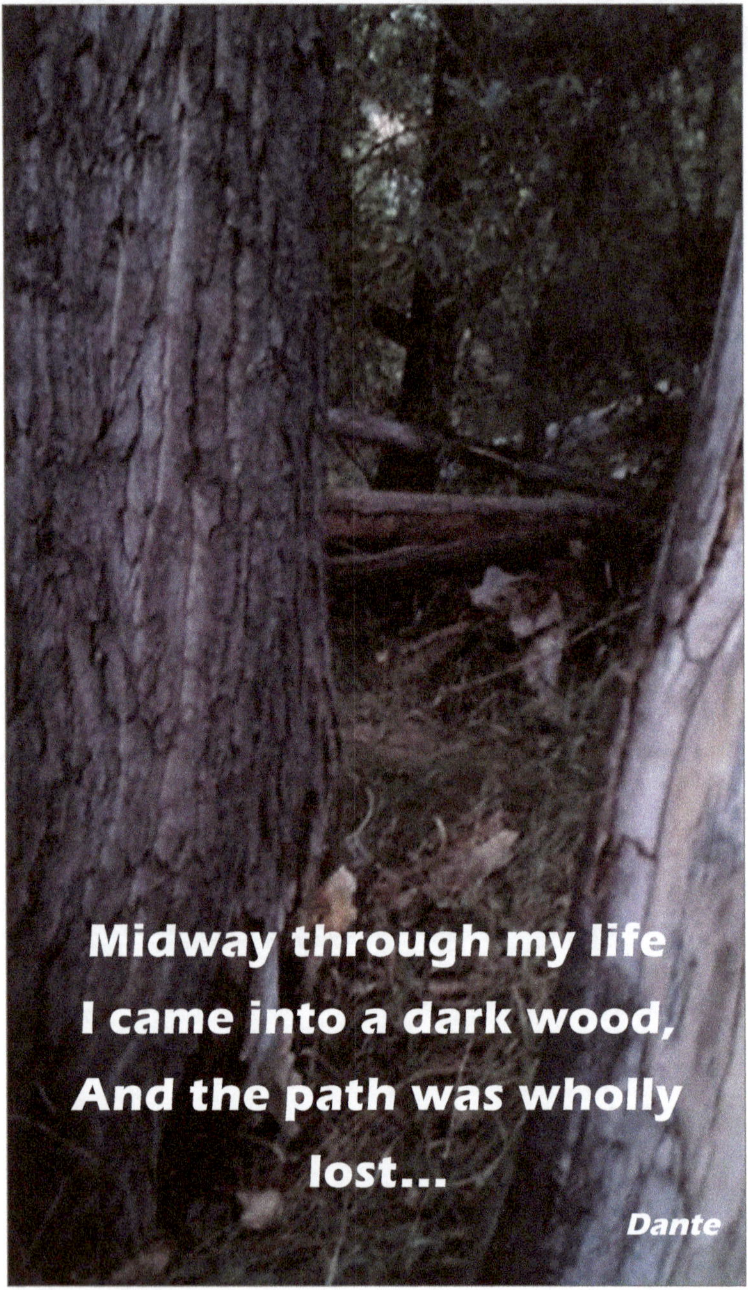
Midway through my life
I came into a dark wood,
And the path was wholly
lost...
Dante

Dark and Forboding Wood by Blair Ashby

Keep Your Fingers On The Wall

In his college days, before he had made himself famous as Mr. Bean and Johnny English, Rowan Atkinson decided he wanted to join the comedic thespian club. The requirement was that he had to make a video of a comedic skit. Based on the video, it would be decided whether he would be accepted, or not. Rowan decided to do an old standard of a distracted man walking into a pole ...but with a twist at the end.

The video shows Rowan walking down the street. Soon he recognizes his friend walking across the street. He waves and gesticulates wildly, trying to get his friend's attention. After a while, a pole enters the scene. Rowan is walking straight towards it. At the very last second, Rowan sees the pole, stops, looks across at his friend all embarrassed, laughs a little bit, waves again, takes two steps around the pole, and falls down a manhole. The video is hilarious and Rowan was accepted into the thespian club.

The video is funny, because life is frequently like this.

You dodge a bullet in a fire fight, only to trip and break your leg on your way to the mess hall.

My dad was trained as a radar technician in the Vietnam war. He was part of a special unit that would sit in towers 50 feet above the jungle canopy monitoring radar that watched Vietcong planes. The vast majority of the guys in his group would never come back because they were sitting targets that high up.

My dad was also a woodworker. While my dad was still in the States, before he shipped out, his commanding officer came to him and asked him to build a bookcase. So my dad went into the Air Force wood shop and started building the bookcase. While sawing the wood, he accidentally cut off three of his fingers. They raced him to the hospital and sewed them back on.

The next day, my dad reported to his CO. The man held up a piece of paper and said, "Ashby, you got lucky this time." He went on, "Here are your orders to ship off for Nam tomorrow," and he ripped the papers up. Was this an accident or a blessing?

My friend Joel was a checkout clerk in a store. He had been there five years. He liked his job and he liked the people. During the last recession, word came through that there were going to be cutbacks. A bunch of the clerks were going to be let go.

Joel caught a rumor that he was going to be transferred to another store, so he felt like everything was okay until he walked into work one day and they handed him a pink slip.

A client of mine, Pat, was working in my studio Friday afternoon. He was looking kind of green. He said he had the flu and he just didn't feel well. I told him to go home and I'd see him Monday morning. Monday morning Pat called me. He said, "I'm not coming in. I may only have a few days left to live. It turns out I don't have the flu, I have very advanced leukemia and my body's failing."

My best friend, Lars, and his wife, Amy, had the exact same model of mobile phone. The two phones were sitting next to each other on an end table when a text came in. Lars, thinking it was his phone, walked over, picked up the phone, opened it up, and it was another man sex-ting his wife. Their marriage ended a few months later.

We've all had friends and colleagues who thought they had perfect kids only to find out that their kids were failing because they had been ditching classes for the past month.

They say an economic down turn is when your neighbor loses his job, a recession is when your spouse loses her job, and a depression is when you lose yours. All of a sudden, for any one of many reasons, you find yourself in the dark.

You are trapped in a pitch-black maze and you have no idea where to go or what to do.

In the middle of March, 2009, three months after my darkness began, a client of mine called me and said he needed some work done. He wanted to do the work late Friday afternoon, so could we meet for lunch. Somewhat confused, I agreed to meet him.

While at lunch, he looked at me and said, “Blair, in the past three or four months, I heard your language change. I’ve seen your actions change. And there is something about me you should know. Before I was a publisher, I was a therapist. And you, you’re in “Midlife.” You’re in clinical depression and you are feeling lost right now.”

With those words, I finally recognized the darkness I had been wallowing in for two and a half months.

I realized that the agony I had been facing had a name, and that meant it was a challenge and that somehow, I could overcome it.

Jim went on to tell me his definition of midlife. He said, “Midlife is when you realize that you are going to die, and you have been fucking around with all kinds of shit for the past twenty years, and you don’t want to fuck around with that shit any more.”

I had to laugh at the definition and at the anger I felt at the darkness that was swallowing me. Yet, now knowing that somehow, I could eventually get out of it.

At that point, Jim went on to tell me that depression is like a pitch-black maze and I remembered the book I'd read about mazes. What most people don't realize is that if you put one hand against one wall of a maze, and you start walking forward, no matter what, eventually you will get out of the maze. You may touch every wall of that maze, and go down every dead end in the maze, but you will get out.

When you are lost in darkness, it is important for you to realize that you have to keep moving forward.

You cannot stand still and wallow in your darkness.

Start walking forward, even if you have no idea where you are going. Keep your hand on the wall and walk.

So now you may be asking, "What is the wall?"

In the early days of your darkness, that wall can generally be defined in only one way: "Not this."

You feel angry. You feel frustrated. You feel trapped. You feel betrayed. This is NOT what you want.

Here's the bottom line. Your old system doesn't work anymore. Whatever model it was, it has failed. You have to shift to a new paradigm, but you have no idea what the new paradigm is, so you feel lost.

It is important for you to realize that you have just started a process of change and growth.

You are shifting gears. But in the process of shifting gears, there is a point where the engine isn't engaged. Sometimes it's okay to coast for a bit and grieve. It's okay to hurt. It's okay to feel angry. It's okay to feel sad. It's okay to feel dark.

But I think it is also important to understand: NOT THIS. You don't want to stay where you are very long, or else the darkness will take over your life.

Just like Rowan Atkinson fell into the manhole, darkness can swallow us up.

During these periods of despair, it's okay to stand where you land, stunned, not quite knowing what's happened.

To feel betrayed, to feel anger, to feel cheated, to feel sad, is okay.

At a certain point, though, you have to start taking control of your life again.

Reach one hand out and touch the wall, knowing that the wall is NOT THIS.

Know, though, that whatever "THIS" is – it's going to be better.

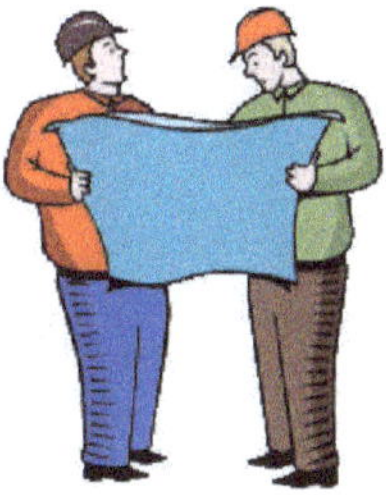

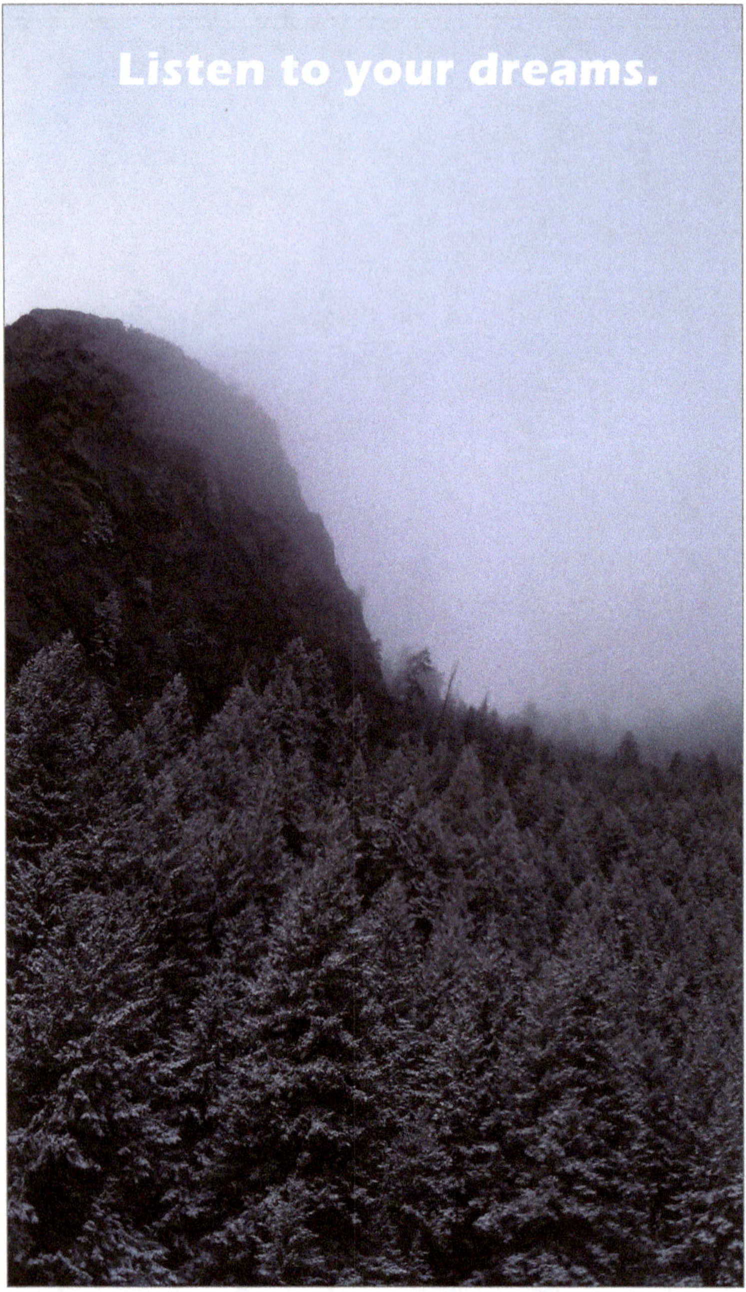

Nederland by Blair Ashby

Feel The Burn...You Are Not What You Feel

Forty-two miles.

My son and I were exactly halfway on the bike trip. We had crossed the city on the river trail from the north end to the south end, riding uphill the whole way. It was pretty hard going. Now we were resting, catching a smoothie to drink, and preparing to tackle the last half.

We started the second half of the journey. The 42 miles in front of us were now downhill.

Strangely, the last half of the journey, even if it is downhill, frequently feels harder.

You're tired. You're achy. You're probably sunburned. And you are certainly not in the mood to be only half-way done.

At around 70 to 72 miles, things started to get rough. We had been riding about five and a half hours by then. My legs hurt. My knees were burning. I frequently felt like my thighs were going to explode. And then, to make matters worse, the wind started to blow directly at us.

So at peak exhaustion, we were riding into the wind. I wanted to give up.

We have all been in these situations before.

Whether it is some kind of sport, or building a house, or buried in a business report, or working on your car, you get to the point where you are sick to death of what you are doing.

The fun is gone and now it is just drudgery as you struggle to reach a goal. Whether that goal is real or perceived doesn't matter.

Here's the ultimate irony. The goal my son and I had that day was to get right back to where we started – our car.

When you're in your darkness, it is frequently your goal too: to get right back to where you started.

You want to return to a place where you aren't feeling this kind of stress. A place where you aren't feeling this kind of anger. A place where you might even have been happy.

Now darkness comes in many forms, shapes, and sizes. It might be anger over losing your job, betrayal by your wife or girlfriend, or sadness over missed dreams and goals left over from your teen years.

No matter what form your darkness takes, you have a choice about how you are going to deal with it.

Your choice comes down to: fight it or be in it. I'll give you a hint though. In the end, you are going to be in it.

You see, you can choose to fight your darkness. And when you fight it, you are like a shadow boxer, except the shadows you're boxing aren't on the wall or the cement floor. They are, in fact, *shadows in your soul, in your mind*.

You can't win. No matter how hard you punch, your fist passes right through them and they don't care. They are still there.

You can deny your darkness by running. But no matter how fast and how far you run, the darkness will catch you. It may not be right away, but it will catch you. And when it does, you will still have to deal with it.

One other option is that maybe you can dodge it. But the darkness never ceases. And if you manage to dodge it for a while, it will circle back around. And when you are least expecting it, it will jump on you again. So . . .

You have a choice. You can fight your darkness or you can be in it.

But at the end of the day, it is going to win. So which are you going to choose? Now, the real question is, why would you spend all your energy fighting it? Part of it is the male mentality. We think we have to fight for what we have.

When I was in my depression, my wife constantly told me to get help. And I constantly told her that I could solve this myself.

She was right. I needed help. But I was not going to give

up that easily. I chose to fight it. In the end, the darkness still won. And a point came when I finally had to accept my defeat and start dealing with the darkness.

When you finally reach that point of surrender, you have new dynamics to move forward into. One of the most important things you have to decide is whether you are going to take an identity from your darkness, or you are just going to be in it.

Let me explain. In the early days of my depression, I used to walk around saying, "I'm depressed."

My friend, Tony, corrected me one day. He said, "Blair, you are not depressed. You feel depression. Don't take an identity from it."

I struggled with that for quite a while until I finally understood one day after smashing my thumb with a hammer. I realized, as I was standing there with my thumb swelling up to the size of a zeppelin, that I was in incredible pain, but I was not THE pain.

This was a watershed moment for me because I finally understood Tony's words.

I am not my depression. I feel depression, but I am not depressed.

As men, we frequently take our identity from our circumstances or emotions.

I have a friend who develops software for a living. When he was laid off, he walked around saying, "I'm a software engineer, and I can't get a job." Because he took his identity from his career and was unemployed, he was having an identity crises. What he does was threatened, thus he felt insecure in himself as well as with his circumstances.

Several months after my divorce, I took a divorce recovery course that lasted ten weeks. During that time, the group would get together once a week and do a bowling night, or a movie night, or a dinner night, or some other activity as a group. After the class was over, many people in the class continued to get together on a weekly basis. Everybody was invited to these activities.

I chose not to go. When I was emailed or called and asked why I wasn't there, I would tell them, "I don't want to hang out with all those divorced people."

Invariably, they would ask, "Why? You're divorced."

And I would say, "No. My marriage ended in divorce. I am not divorced."

This simple act of a language change helped me find my identity as something inside of me, not something pertaining to my circumstances or emotions.

Once you can see your darkness as something you feel, and you can accept your darkness as a feeling you are having and not a definition of who you are, you can start to be in it.

Like I mentioned in an earlier section, at sometime when you were younger, you may have built some dreams about how you wanted your life to be. Then slowly you started to make little compromises to accomplish shorter term goals until you sacrificed the longer term dream that you had.

Whenever you would make one of these sacrifices, your dream would whisper into your ear, "Hey, what about me?"

Now, if you were anything like me, you ignored the voice. You had short term goals to accomplish with results that could be seen right away. The rewards were quick and easy, so you made even more sacrifices. Doing a little bit more here. Working a little bit more there.

Each time you did, your dream would say a little bit louder, "Hey, what about me?"

As you kept ignoring that dream, it would get more violent in its approach.

It would start to yell. And then it would scream. And then it would throw a rock at you. Eventually it would start hitting you with a stick, yelling, "What about me?"

When you still didn't pay attention to your dream, it would nuclear bomb you with depression and darkness.

The minute you decide to surrender to your darkness and be in it, you take the first step toward walking out of it.

What I am telling you is that your darkness may, in fact, be you trying to get your attention about your life. If you are shadow boxing with your darkness, you are fighting yourself.

Being in your darkness gives your dream an opportunity to talk to you.

Chances are, you are not going to like what the dream you have ignored so long has to say, but it's important that you listen.

And that is why being in your darkness is so vital. As you sit in the darkness, you start to look around at it. You start to understand it. You're a man! You start trying to figure it out.

Take this time to describe your darkness to yourself. Take this time to understand what you are feeling. Take this time to see how your darkness reacts to the things in your life.

When you're ready, my suspicion is that you will begin to understand why you are feeling this darkness. And that is a major step in leaving the darkness.

When you can ask yourself, "Why am I feeling so angry? Why am I feeling so betrayed? Why am I feeling so down?" you can begin to assess the motivations underneath the darkness. Those motivations are probably your dreams trying to talk with you.

This will probably take a long time. It is not easy. You have to be willing to listen to a lot of self-criticism about how you've lived your life up to this point.

It's like standing in front of a mirror naked. You are never quite happy with what you see.

Being in your darkness at this time is a way to learn from it. It's a way to learn from you. It's a way to learn about you. It's a way to learn about the things you have sacrificed and about the things you have gained; about what things are really worth to you and what things aren't worth so much to you.

It is a period of hard lessons when you have to be willing to accept things and know that you could have done some things better, but you did them the best you could at the time, with the knowledge that you had.

Your darkness is a chance to increase your knowledge. It is a chance to learn about you.

Listen to your dreams. Listen to what they are telling you. Listen to your failings, and listen to your successes.

Most importantly, just be in your darkness and listen to yourself.

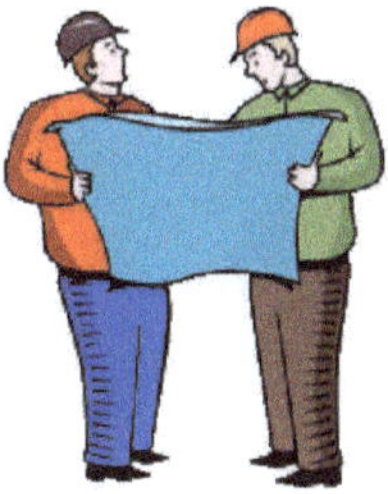

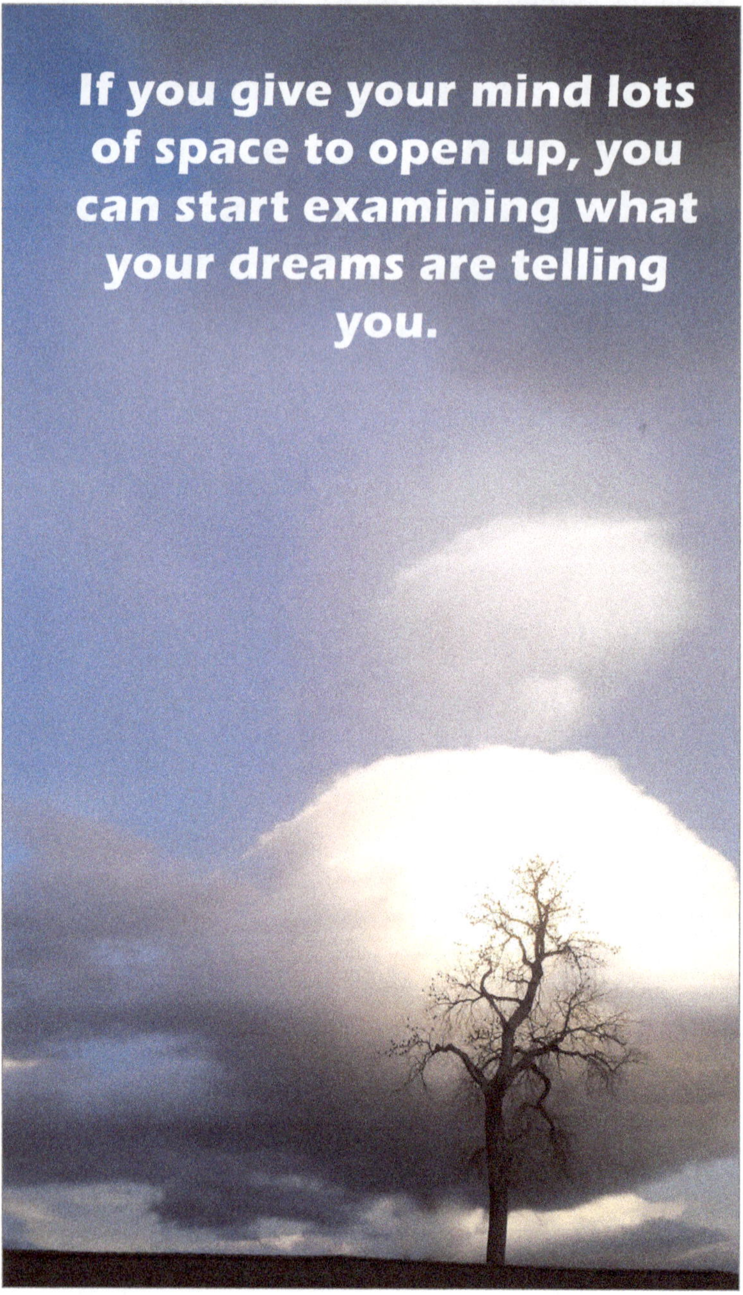
If you give your mind lots of space to open up, you can start examining what your dreams are telling you.

Tree and Cloud by Blair Ashby

Shut Up! And Listen To Yourself

A couple of months ago, I was sitting in a restaurant talking with a friend. I was complaining about a situation and the frustration I was feeling trying to get it worked out my way.

All of a sudden, she interrupted me. She said, "Blair. Shut up! And listen to yourself."

She went on to explain that my problem with the whole situation had nothing to do with the circumstances. But in fact, it had to do with my attitude about the circumstances.

The situation was worth complaining about. There were some issues that had to be addressed. But what I was doing was actually trying to cross bridges that hadn't even been built yet. I was wasting energy worrying about things that didn't exist.

What I really needed to do, was to deal with the issue at hand and not worry about imaginary realities that didn't exist.

Probably the most humorous thing about the whole situation was that I actually knew a solution to the whole circumstance and was talking about it. But because I hadn't thought it through, and wasn't listening to myself, I couldn't see it.

Thus, when Kira said to me, "Blair, shut up and listen to yourself," what in fact she was saying was: You already know the answer. You just aren't getting it.

When you are dealing with darkness, it is frequently the same way.

You already know the answer. You just aren't hearing yourself.

In the previous section, I talked a little bit about listening to your dreams.

Now, the dreams I am talking about are not the dreams at night-time, and they are not some ethereal, new age-y thing.

I am talking about the goals you had set for your life that quite possibly you aren't meeting or living up to. I'm a firm believer that these dreams will get your attention in some way or another. Frequently, if you don't listen, they will get your attention by bringing darkness upon you.

That means, when you listen to your dreams, you are actually listening to yourself, talking to yourself about the areas in your life which you need to work on or improve.

Have you ever noticed that when you are doing your favorite hobby or activity, your brain tends to shut off and focus exclusively on that project or activity? It's almost as if all the noise that surrounds and fills our lives all the time goes away when we are concentrating on that activity or hobby.

And that is exactly what happens. Your brain gets so caught up focusing, it shuts out everything else.

Now, let's take it a step further. Have you ever noticed that often times, when you are focusing on something really intently, that is when you find the solution to another problem completely unrelated to what you are focusing on.

So you might be focusing intently on your draft picks for your fantasy football team, when all of a sudden, the solution to a problem that has been vexing you at work pops into your head.

What is really happening is that you have created space for your brain to work on things besides all the noise that's flooding into it.

Find something to concentrate on, even when you are feeling your lowest.

When I was in the midst of my deepest depression, I walked. I would walk anywhere from three to twelve miles a day. During this time, by keeping my feet busy moving forward one step at a time, I gave my mind lots of space to open up and start examining what my dreams were telling me.

Your point of concentration can be anything:

- Playing basketball
- Working on your car
- Renovating your house
- Gardening
- Hunting and/or fishing
- Meditating
- Working out
- Running marathons
- Anything that requires your focus

Whatever it is for you, it doesn't matter.

Focus exclusively on your activity so you can free your mind to deal with the deeper issues without you having to concentrate on them directly.

There is a story about a prophet named Elijah. Elijah managed to really irritate the ruler of the land, so much so that a death warrant was put out on his head. Elijah took off into the wilderness to hide. He found a mountain that had a cave in it, so he hiked in and decided to camp out there for a while.

The story goes, that one afternoon, he was sitting in the mouth of the cave when a powerful windstorm came through. It was so powerful, in fact, that the story says that the mountains were split and rocks were shattered.

Then the earth began to shake. An earthquake came along and flattened another portion of the mountain. Lastly, a fire came through and burned everything that was left to a cinder. Elijah was left overlooking a pretty decimated mountainside. The story ends by saying that after these three horrific events, a still small voice came and spoke to Elijah, giving him instruction on how to move forward.

Now, if we imagine our daily lives and how many distractions we have, it is pretty easy to equate the noise of all these disasters happening to Elijah (windstorms, earthquakes, wildfires) with all the noise we face on a daily basis in our reality. Add to that noise, the blackness of your soul, and you're in darkness. This equates quite well to the black earth that was left after fires scorched Elijah's mountain.

The essential point to all this is after the noise, after the destruction, Elijah heard a still small voice that re-empowered him to move out and take control of his life. And that is the same thing that can happen to you.

When you are sitting in all the destruction, all the darkness going on in your life, if you take time to just shut up and listen to yourself, you can start to hear your dreams – that still small voice trying to reach out to you.

And that is where your hobby or activity comes into play. The more you focus on your hobby, the more you are able to give your dream space in your mind to talk to you.

You can be busy shooting hoops while your brain is working through the issues that are bringing the darkness into your life.

If you are, instead, distracting your brain with television, or podcasts, or movies, or surfing the web, or working relentlessly all the time, then there is no space in your brain for your dreams to talk to you.

In eastern philosophies, they call this busy-ness in our heads, the chattering mind.

I know, in my skull, that is pretty accurate. Frequently, I will go over and over a conversation or hammer through events relentlessly, trying to get to some kind of conclusion that doesn't exist until I sit back and let my subconscious take over.

Sitting back and letting your subconscious take over takes practice.

I have to be willing to focus on whatever activity I am doing, whether it is composing a song or writing a chapter in this book or mowing my field, and just let my dreams do the work in the background.

When I was in my depression, the way I did this was on long walks. I would take anywhere from one to five walks a day. Each one would be three or four miles long. I went through four pairs of tennis shoes one summer that way.

On these walks, I would start out by going over, and over, and over again all the noise in my mind, all the darkness and anger and depression I was feeling.

However, I found that after walking for half an hour or 45 minutes, my mind started to quiet and I could just walk.

I stopped thinking. I stopped chattering. I stopped doing anything except walking.

And that's when I started to make headway on the real darkness inside of me. Instead of focusing on the darkness, I started listening to the still small voice that was whispering, "Hey, what about me."

It took me months of walking before I started to feel like I was making some progress. It took a lot of practice. And when I say that it took a lot of practice, for me, that means I had to keep walking. Fortunately for me, that was easy. The walking brought some relief from the depression and the anxiety that was racing through my body all the time.

My suspicion is that whatever you find is your activity, it will be the same way. It'll be something that gives you a small amount of relief from the darkness and the suffering you are going through.

That kind of distraction is good. It's not adding noise to your life. It's adding quietness.

So find an activity, preferably a healthy one. Make sure it is one you do alone. Don't have yourself surrounded by your friends distracting you with more noise. Spend time in that activity. Work at it. Practice at it.

Whatever it is you choose to do, spend a lot of time in that activity, focusing your brain on it, so your dreams can focus on you.

While you're doing that activity, feel free to think about the darkness and feel free to think about your dreams. That's okay. It's the fact that you are concentrating on something else that really helps this process.

There is a fantastic jazz album written by Madonna's producer. The whole album is dedicated to fly fishing. Fly fishing became the activity that Patrick Leonard used to concentrate his mind and to distract himself from all the noise in his life. It's almost a religion to him. Not like a church religion, but it is somewhat a spiritual retreat. And that's what your activity needs to be for you.

In my case it was walking several times a day that gave me the time to start dealing with the darkness. In your case, whatever activity your choose, doing that activity every day or several times a week will be you starting to walk out of your darkness.

It will be you starting to take control of your life again.

It will be you starting to chase your dreams. It will be you making your life happen your way.

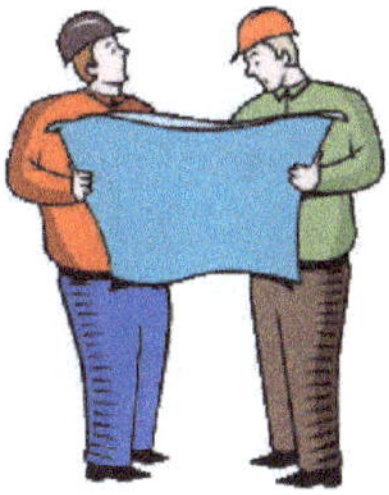

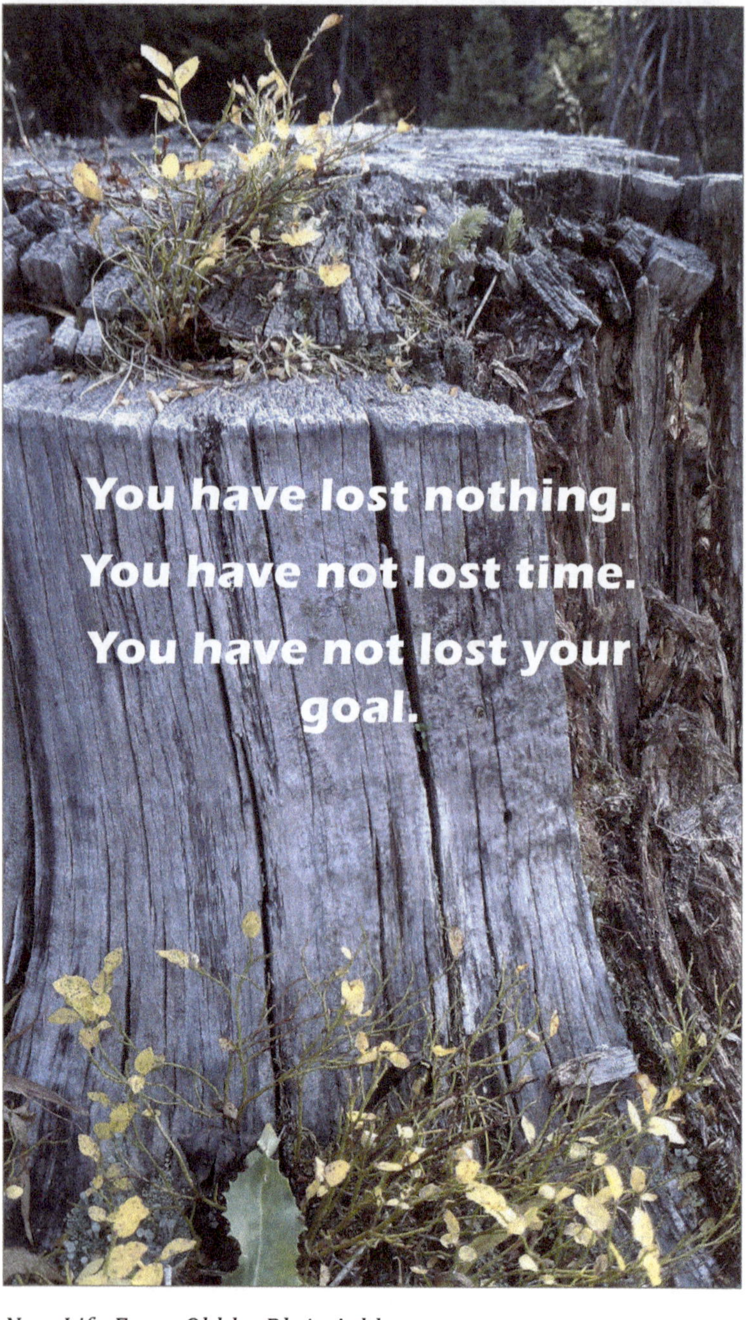
You have lost nothing.
You have not lost time.
You have not lost your goal.

New Life From Old by Blair Ashby

Epiphanies Take Time

This was one of the hardest tools for me to learn during my time of depression. The last thing I wanted to hear when I was in my darkness was that:

- Answers don't come quick, or
- I may have to be in this misery for a while, or
- The best path out of this misery isn't necessarily the fast one.

This is not encouraging news when you are sitting in darkness. And so, it was one of the most difficult tools for me to learn.

I never wanted to be in darkness to begin with. I never wanted to suffer from depression. So why did I have to wait for this to be fixed? Especially when people are telling me that I have to wait on me to deal with my stuff. And that is the only way I'm going to fix this.

My thought was, "That's a load of crap and I don't want to hear that stuff."

I felt like I was a victim here when, in fact, I wasn't.

This was just my dreams trying to get a hold of me. But I didn't see it that way, yet. And that was one of the main epiphanies. It took some time for me to get it.

One evening, during the writing of this book, I was sitting in my favorite pizza parlor with my parents and I was talking with my dad about this section. I was getting his opinion on how he thought I should word this so that it would be general enough for everyone, and specific enough for anyone suffering from darkness.

My dad and I were batting around ideas when, all of a sudden, the universe solved this in one easy step. The "step" was approximately 6'2" and a young 20-something man.

He was wearing shorts with the down-around-your-butt look but he was taking this fad and accelerating it to new levels of ridiculousness. He didn't have one pair of shorts hanging down around his butt, he had two.

He looked like some overly ambitious stapler had gone crazy in his laundry basket and this guy had pulled on his shorts in the morning without bothering to find out what it looked like. He had his boxers, then he had a middle pair of shorts. Over that he had an outer pair of shorts. The outer pair of shorts were hanging all the way below his butt, and the middle pair of shorts were half-way up his butt-cheeks. The outer pair appeared to be stapled to the middle pair and the middle pair appeared to be stapled to his boxer shorts so this whole contraption would stay up on him.

It looked incredibly stupid. But he couldn't see that yet.

This is one of those things that five years from now, he is going to look at pictures of himself that his friends took and he is going to think, "Wow, it was really stupid to wear my shorts that way."

And ten years from now, when he's an early 30-something, he is going to look at that picture, and he's going to be truly embarrassed and say, "Wow, I looked like a dork."

Ten to fifteen years from now, when he is between 30 and 35, he is finally going to realize: "I was so busy being caught up in looking like part of the herd that I completely forgot to pay attention to myself and my self-respect."

This will be a major epiphany to him when he can finally accept that he was foolish enough to follow the herd and not stand up for himself. I suspect he will be so embarrassed, he will condemn himself for his actions. But this realization will take time – I'm estimating 10 to 15 years for him to get it.

This is a great example of . . .

Epiphanies take time.

My dad is a retired cabinet maker. He did beautiful work. Sometime, when he was around 35 to 40 years old, he was lifting a 900 pound counter top into a truck with a little bit of help when he realized that in 20 years he wouldn't want to be doing this kind of hard work anymore.

It took him 15 more years to come up with a business plan that allowed him to move into a fantastic company selling wholesale kitchen cabinets.

Epiphanies take time, and once you put the idea out there, you have to wait on them to materialize.

Now here is an encouragement that I want to give you: If you are in darkness now, it is quite likely that you have already had that epiphany. You just haven't realized it yet.

At some point in your past – 5 years, 10 years, 15 years, or 20 years ago – you realized something. You realized that you weren't going after your dreams and goals which you thought you had been going after.

When my dad was 40-something, he realized he was working too hard. At 50 years old, he had to go through a realignment to get his goals and priorities straight so he could chase after his real dream which was, "I don't want to work this hard." That was the dream that he had first put out 10 or 15 years earlier when he was lifting a 900 pound counter top.

If you remember, in one of the earlier tools, I talked about how, when you make a small sacrifice of your dream, your dream whispers, "Hey, what about me?"

Well, this darkness is now your dream screaming in your

ears, "HEY! WHAT ABOUT ME?"

If you're experiencing that, you've probably already had that epiphany. You just didn't realize it.

So what you need to start doing is looking in the darkness for that dream. You need to start examining it and figure out what it is, where it is.

This is painful stuff, because you have to look at these things and ask, "When and why did I take the wrong fork in the road that sacrificed my long term goals for short term, easy gains?"

Like I said in the last tool, you have to address some of the failing you have done in your life. But once you get through that part, then you can start to see your reality clearly, and start to make adjustments and alignments to shape your reality the way you want it to be.

You can begin to take back your life.

I spent fourteen months in depression because I refused to deal with the fact that I had missed some of my dreams. And it was my fault.

My depression was my dreams and my goals coming back and saying, "HEY! WHAT ABOUT ME?"

Once I started to acknowledge that, I started to examine the darkness and question why. I could start looking at that "HEY! WHAT ABOUT ME?" and examining what my dreams were actually saying.

They were saying things like, "Hey, you missed your goal

back in 1995 by getting distracted and chasing after the short-term reward. Now it's time to realign your life and start chasing those goals again."

It's not too late! You can accomplish those things. In fact, all the knowledge that you now have will make it an even more effective goal than you had before.

That is maybe the most important part of this tool.

You have not failed up to this point. You have lived your life the best you could live it. Now, though, you have options.

The universe is giving you a chance to realign your life your way. You need to take advantage of it.

This is when you can look at all the experiences you have garnered in the last 5, 10, 15, 20 years, and piece it together so you can put together your life your way.

You can learn from your experiences. You can build upon the foundation that you've already created. You have lost nothing. You have not lost time. You have not lost your goal.

In fact, one way to look at this is that the universe felt that you needed to learn the things you have learned in your past so you're ready at this point to realign your life your way.

It really is okay that it's taken this long.

As you feel the burn from the darkness you're sitting in,

and as you shut up and shut off the noise in your life and listen to yourself, have the expectation that epiphanies take some time. Be patient. You are going to get answers that will help you move into a life that is happy and fulfilling for you.

Part of all this is just the process of walking through it. That is where you're at right now. As Winston Churchill said, "When you are going through hell, keep going."

So take this time to:

- Listen to yourself and learn
- Hear yourself and understand
- Ask yourself "why?"

Then take those answers to those questions and build the life you really want to live. Because . . .

After you walk out of this darkness, you are going to live a fuller life than you could ever imagine.

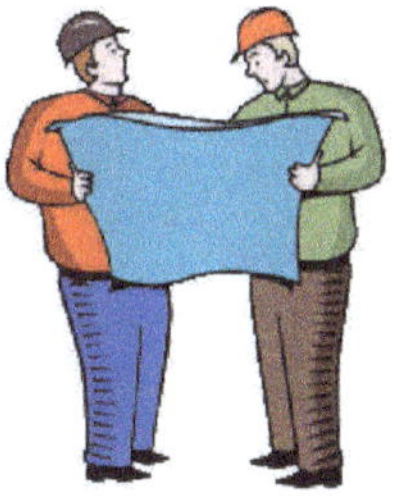

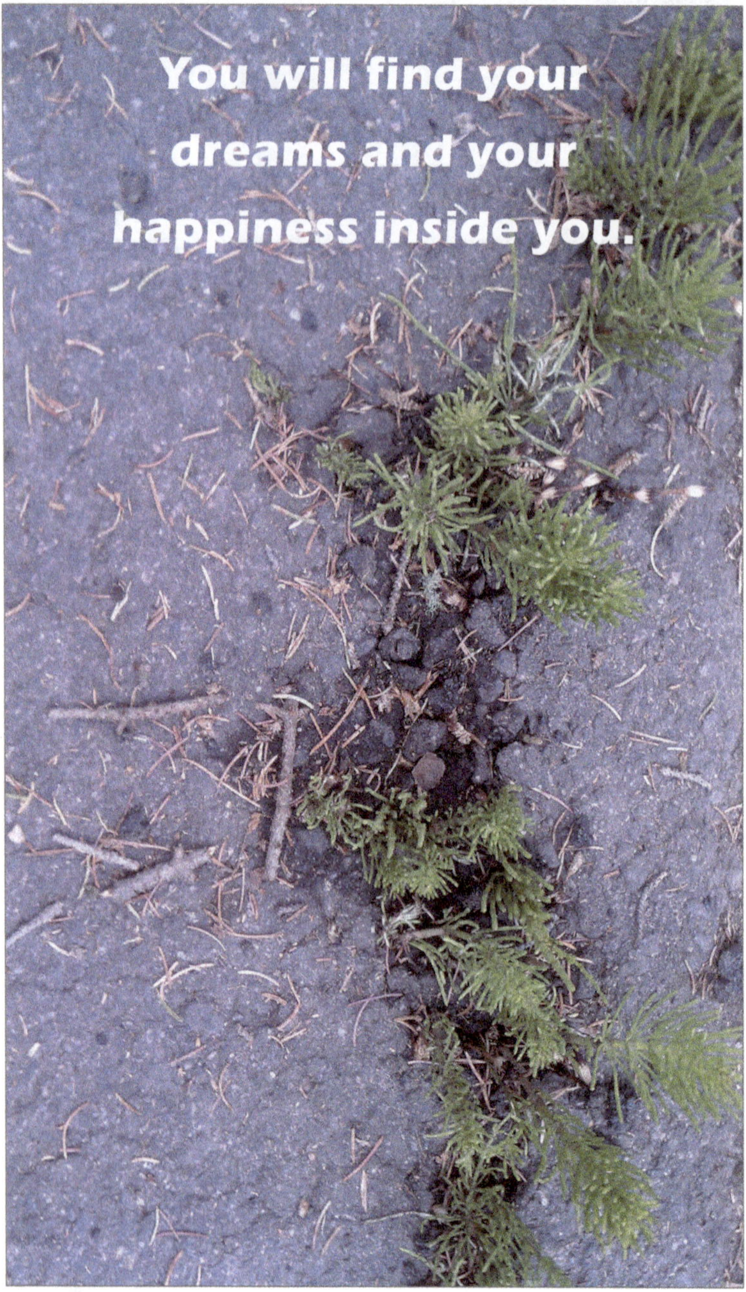
You will find your
dreams and your
happiness inside you.

Trees In Paving by Blair Ashby

You Gotta Grow On

Greg and I were driving into the mountains, heading to a trail head to spend the day hiking. We were talking about change and crisis and our own personal experience with these realities.

Just as I was driving around a corner on a canyon road and we were getting ready to head into a tunnel, Greg said something that was so simple, yet so profound, that I actually had to stop for a minute and process it.

He said, "Isn't crisis just the realization that you've grown too big for your skin? And just like a snake has to rub through nooks and crannies to shed it's old skin, that is what crisis requires of us."

Wow. That brings it into clarity in a hurry.

To grow and improve our lives, we frequently have to let go of the old ways that hold us back.

That is especially true if we have deep attachments to those old ways.

When Abraham Lincoln was elected president, he had

to let go of peaceful solutions to the dilemma of human rights.

When Hitler attacked Poland, Europe had to let go of the concept of the "Great War" (World War I) being the last world war.

When NASA wanted to land on the moon, they had to let go of the concept of the pilot sitting down, and convert the lunar modules to standing so that the astronauts knees could absorb the impact of the landing.

Part of growth is letting go of the things that are holding you back.

When I was 20 and at university, I was in a communication class and it was speech day. Now I love public speaking, and I had prepared for this. I had my note cards and I was ready to go. What I had failed to anticipate was the speech prior to mine.

Shawn got up and talked about cocaine addiction and watching his brother's life wither away to death through an addiction to cocaine. The story was heavy and profound and it was sad. The class of about 50 students was stunned into silence when it ended.

Unfortunately, the schedule the professor had put up

required each speech to start one minute (give or take) after the previous speech so that everybody could fit into the time allotted. There was no time to let the audience decompress.

I walked up, stood in front of the class, and realized all of my preparation was for naught. The speech I had planned to give would fail miserably. I had to come up with something in a hurry and on the fly.

So I picked my note cards off the podium, threw them over my shoulder, and proceeded to say, "Do remember when Luke was flying through the equator of the Death Star? He brought his weapon's guidance down and was preparing to take the 'winning shots' when a little voice said to him, 'Use the force, Luke. Use the force.' Luke shut down the guidance system and went on intuition. We know the end of the story. The Death Star was destroyed and there was a great celebration."

That broke the negative trance that held the audience after the previous speech and allowed me to go ahead and give a truncated version of my prepared speech.

I don't think it would have worked, though, if I hadn't been willing to throw all my preparation away and start fresh.

Your darkness is exactly the same.

You have road blocks to improving your life.

You have some old programs, some old ways of doing things, or thinking about things. You have old methods which you employ.

Part of walking out of the darkness is being willing to let go of the things that brought you into the darkness to begin with.

I realize that may sound funny. "Why, wouldn't I let go of things that have been a problem for me?" You might ask.

But the fact is, the saying frequently holds true: Better the devil you know than the devil you don't.

We men sometimes find it easier to continue going the wrong way rather than asking directions or searching out new ways to do it better.

Just look at the stereotype of a man who is lost and isn't going to ask for directions or examine the map. He 'knows' he can figure it out himself. You have to let go of that kind of mentality if you're going to get un-lost.

Walking through your own personal valley of the shadow of death is the same way.

In the previous sections, I have talked about sitting and listening to your darkness and crisis and learning from it. I've spoken of examining it and trying to understand why it is happening to you.

This tool makes the assumption that you have started to learn something from that examination.

Now you need to let go of some of those things that put

you in darkness to begin with.

You need to understand what you've learned and grow on.

Paganini was a super-star composer and violinist in the 1800s. He got a contract to play a few gigs at the French conservatory in Paris. Just like the big rock stars of today, with guitar techs and drum techs to take care of their instruments, Paganini had a violin tech. He and the violin tech took two separate trains to Paris.

When Paganini arrived in Paris, the conductor met him at the train station and said, "Paganini, where is your violin?"

Paganini said, "The tech's got it. He'll be bringing it later." When the tech arrived, Paganini met him at the train station along with the conservatory conductor. And, there was no violin.

The tech looked at Paganini and said, "I thought you had the violin."

Paganini said, "I thought you had it."

The conservatory conductor proceeded to have a melt down and go only slightly out of his mind.

"Don't worry," Paganini assured him, "It will work out."

Later that day, as they were walking to the conservatory for the concert, they passed a small boy on the street corner playing a violin. He had his hat out to collect donations.

Paganini offered the boy 500 francs to use his violin for the evening. That was a lifetime's wages for some people in those days. The boy, of course, said yes, and handed Paganini his violin.

The newspapers of the day report that concert was the finest Paganini had ever played. The critics raved about it for the next week.

After the show, as the music conductor was walking Paganini back to the train station, he asked, "How did you do it? How did you play such an amazing concert on a piece of junk violin?"

Paganini looked at him and said, "My dear man, don't you realize, the music is in the Paganini. It's not in the violin."

At some point, Paganini realized that his excellent Stradivarius violin was not the source of the beautiful music that came out of it. It was something deep in his soul that spoke musically. That voice in his soul was his dream.

You are the same way. Whatever it is that you really, really, really want, that is your dream.

It is not your tools. It is not your career. It is not your fancy car. It is not your fancy house. It is not your perfect vacation or your perfect wife or your perfect kids. It is not any of these things that make you happy. It is living your dream that makes you happy.

The dream you have inside you is intrinsic to you. If you are happy (or not) is intrinsic to you, too.

Letting go of the thought that the perfect job, the perfect car, the perfect house, the perfect wife, the perfect kids will make you happy is one extremely important stage of letting go of your darkness and walking into a more happy life.

It is not about changing your external circumstances to fit your thoughts of what you think will make you happy. Rather, it is about transforming your internal processes and finding the happiness inside of you . . . no matter what your situation is.

You've got to grow on.

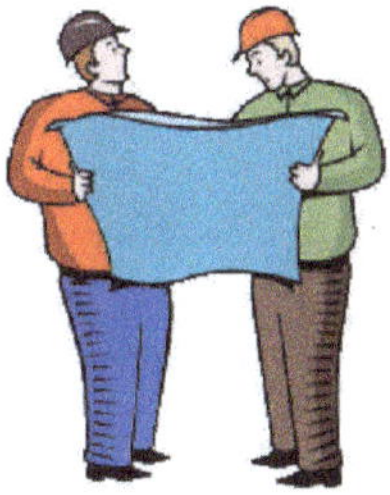

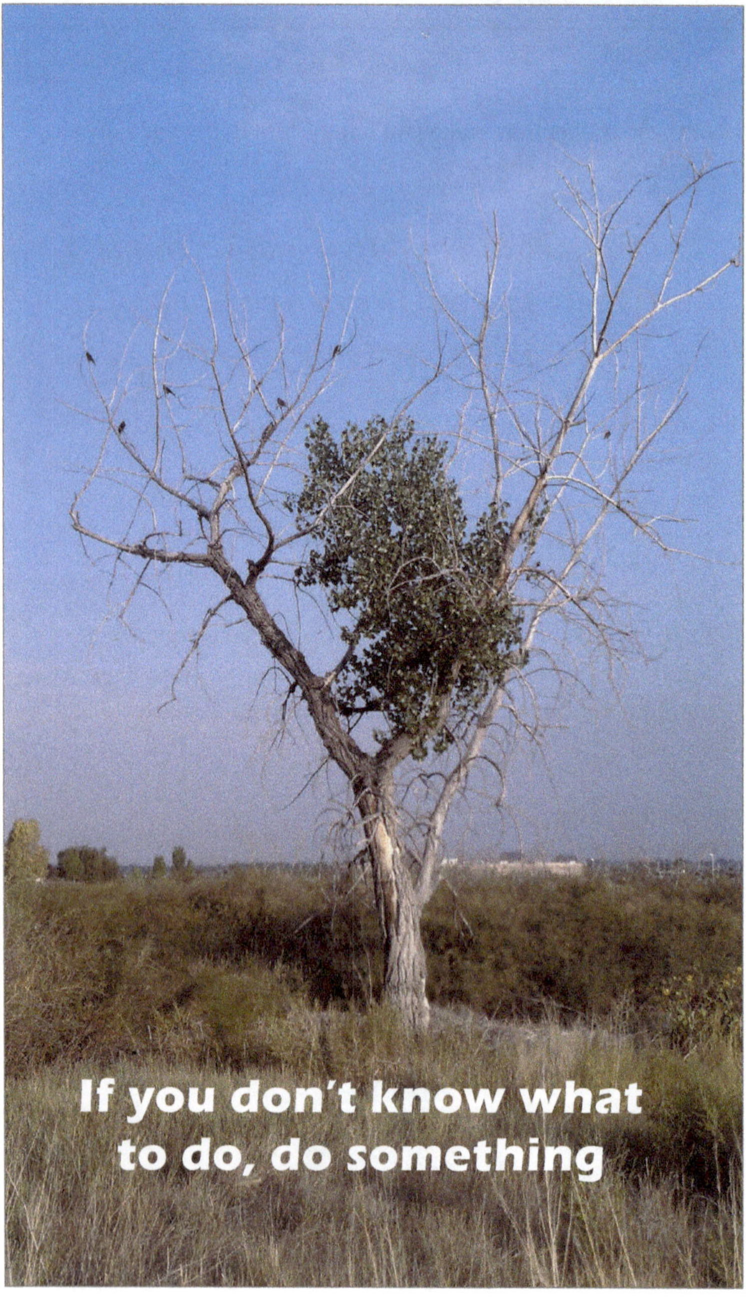

Dead Alive Tree by Blair Ashby

Just Do Something

(a story)

An old man lived up on a mountain with a fresh spring beside his house. The spring ran a few paces away from the house and then disappeared back into the mountain.

Some distance below his house, the old man had a small garden. At the foot of the garden there was a path used by hikers.

Every morning, the old man carried a bucket of water to the garden to water the sparse plants, but he struggled day to day to feed himself on the very little that would grow at his lofty altitude.

One day, a new man stopped by to visit. The old man offered the new man a small bite to eat and some fresh mountain spring water to drink.

With gratitude, the new man took the morsel of food and the large cup of water. He drank a large gulp and then chewed slowly the small morsel, after which he drank deeply again from the large cup.

The old man watched in a sad silence for he had very little food to share.

When the new man had finished, he looked at the old man and asked him why he had only offered a small morsel of food to eat yet so much water to drink.

The old man said, "I can not grow more than that, for the altitude prevents my plants from growing."

The new man said, "But you have so much water!"

The old man said, "I have unlimited water, but even if I watered the plants to saturation, they don't grow for the altitude is too high for them to thrive."

The new man said, "What do you do to help the growing happen?"

The old man said, "Nothing I do matters, so I do nothing. I have lost my will to work the garden for it provides me no reward."

The new man paused and then said, "You have so much water, maybe you should just do something." And with that last statement, he left the old man's house.

The next morning, the old man got up and thought about the new man's words: "Just do something."

The old man put one bucket of water on the plants.

The second morning, the new man's words echoed in his mind again. So the old man went out and put two buckets of water on the garden instead of one. The garden soil got muddy.

The third day, the old man put three buckets of water on the garden, the fourth day four, and so on.

Soon, all that happened was that the soil got saturated and the water started to pool at the base of the garden beside the path.

On the seventh day, after seven buckets of water, the old man noticed two hikers had stopped at the pool which had formed at the bottom of the garden by the path.

"Hello," he said to the two hikers.

They looked up at him and said, "We've been hiking for many hours. We are hot and tired. This pool of water looks so refreshing! May we have a drink and wash our faces?"

"Gladly," said the old man and he went inside to rest. Several hours later, he came back out to check the garden.

Sitting beside the pool was a fresh loaf of bread with a note that said, "Thank you for the water. Here is a gift to show our appreciation."

The eighth day, eight buckets. Ninth day, nine buckets. Each day, there were more hikers and more gifts of appreciation. On the tenth day, the old man got an idea: "I want food to eat. I have unlimited water. Maybe I could trade water for food . . ."

On the eleventh day, the old man dug a trench at the top of the garden and rerouted the spring into it. Now his garden was watered automatically and the pool at the base grew and freshened up.

Hikers stopped by regularly and the old man set up a stall to collect gifts and make trades.

One day, months later, the new man stopped at the stall. The old man looked up and said, "You were right! I just had to do something!"

The new man said, "Yes. When we lose our strength and will for life, sometimes just doing something we need to do opens the way for new ideas to happen. Our forced motivations can sometimes become our desired inspirations."

Even if you don't know what your dream is, do something aimed at your interests! Because even if it's not a perfect fit, you'll learn from it and move towards what's better.

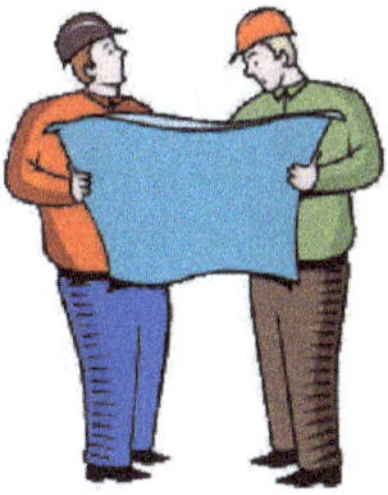

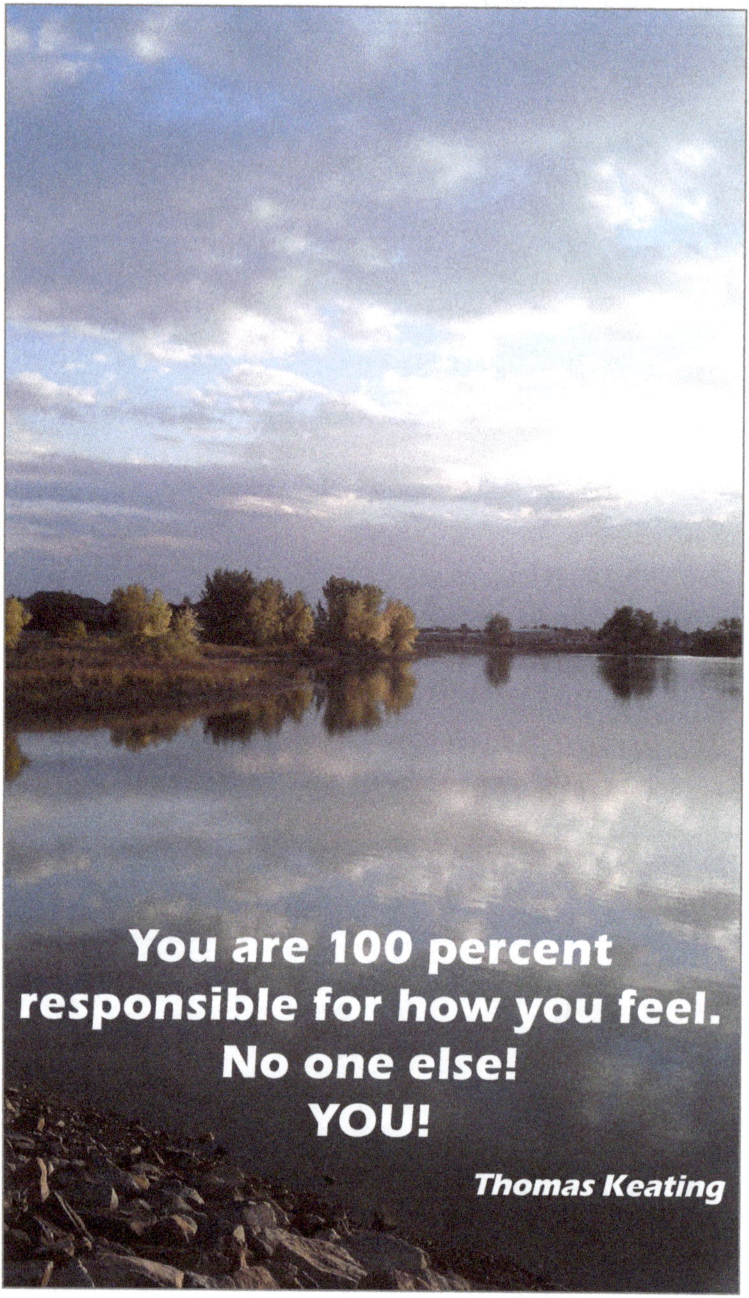
You are 100 percent
responsible for how you feel.
No one else!
YOU!
Thomas Keating

McKay Lake Tree Reflection by Blair Ashby

Deal With Your Stuff

I had been in depression for 12 months when circumstances made it obvious to me I needed to seek therapy.

Depression for me was an evil vice that squeezed the life out of everything and disconnected me from all that was going on around me.

Even on the brightest sun-shiny days, the world was dark and a pervasive charcoal mist covered everything around me.

I struggled to stay connected to myself as much as to my family and the world I lived in.

Depression and darkness for you probably takes on a different form. Whatever form it takes, it is probably just as dark, just as terrifying, just as horrible, and just as maniacal as anything I experienced.

Your darkness is a beast unto itself and no one can truly understand the reality you're living in when you're in that darkness.

Most of the time, I expect, you feel alone. But you need to

understand, you are not truly alone.

There are people available to help you.

My first therapist was a little gal who I chose because she wasn't threatening to me. Quite the statement for a man who could fix it all himself, huh?

At the end of our fourth session, she told me she was thinking about referring me to another therapist. At the end of our fifth session, she gave me the name of another therapist and said she felt I would be better served by him. So, a week later, I sat in his waiting room wondering why she referred me.

Tom greeted me and invited me into his office. It was big. It had a bookshelf all along one wall, full of books. It had two comfortable fabric couches in an L-formation, two easy chairs, and an enormous desk.

As I sat on the couch looking around, I swear, Tom was looking at me with glee as he metaphorically strapped on steel toed boots.

Tom asked me a question, and I started to talk. I talked about the depression I was feeling. I talked about my marriage which was failing. I talked about the lousy economy, and I talked about how unhappy I was.

Tom looked at me and he said, "Blair, what's your part in this?"

Now a few weeks earlier, a client of mine had been in the studio and in talking about his mid-life crisis, he said one of the hardest things he had to deal with was, "What's my shit."

So I looked at Tom, chuckled, and said, "Oh, you're asking me what's my shit."

Tom looked at me and said, "It's time to deal with you, Blair."

We men have a tendency to blame anything else for our issues. We don't think anything is our fault.

For the next four sessions, I complained about people or situations and he said, "Blair, that's their issue. Now, what about you?" Sometime between the fourth and the fifth session, though, I started to get it.

The final drive to write this book and to start talking about these issues was initiated by Ted. (Ted was one of my clients. I had worked for him for about 15 years and felt I knew him pretty well.)

About eight months before writing this book, Ted walked into my studio an angry and bitter man. He proceeded to give me an earful about a business partnership he'd had for two decades and how his partner was messing everything up.

He yelled about everything his partner did wrong, everything his partner said wrong, and how angry and tired he was of dealing with his partner and all his stuff.

He went on to say, the next day he was going to set his partner down, yell, holler, and scream about everything his partner had done wrong, and let his partner know how lousy his partner had been.

I asked Ted if yelling was going to encourage his partner to stay in their partnership. He said probably not, but he needed to get that stuff out anyway.

Without telling Ted I was doing this, I encouraged him to yell for another 10 or 15 minutes about his partner. And he did.

It was nothing specific and it was nothing personal. It was mainly about how angry and mad Ted was. It was about Ted.

After Ted had yelled out a bunch of his energy, I quietly asked him if he would consider another course of action.

Thankfully, for his partnership, Ted said yes.

I asked Ted to go home, look in the mirror, and ask himself these questions:

- "What is my stuff?"
- "What am I doing that is wrong?"
- "What am I doing that is making things worse?"
- "What am I doing that is contributing to the lousy situation?"
- (And most important) "What can I do to improve myself?"

I then told him that as he started to deal with his stuff, for the next couple of months things with his partner would probably get worse, not better.

I went on to tell him to be patient and continually work on improving himself – to constantly deal with his stuff.

A month before writing this book, Ted called and asked to meet me. Two days later, over drinks, Ted told me that he had done everything I had advised and that he and his partner had enjoyed the most productive summer in years.

He went on to say that, sure enough, the first two months had been worse, not better. But pretty soon, his partner started responding to Ted's improvements. His partner started to improve without Ted ever having to say anything.

Eventually, Ted and his partner got to a place where they could talk about their respective issues and deal with them on a mature, non-emotional level.

This is just one example of dealing with your stuff.

In my life, I had to acknowledge all the little things I had done at the expense of my bigger goals.

My wife was always number one to me but she felt like she played second to my career. My goal of being a music producer was frequently sacrificed to the smaller goals of making enough money for a small goal versus the bigger one, and on and on.

My therapist, Tom, brought me to a point where I had to look at myself. I had to look at my responsibility for why my life wasn't going my way.

Thomas Keating has said many times: You are 100 percent responsible for how you feel. No one else! YOU!

I add to that: If you're feeling a negative emotion about something, ask yourself why you feel that way. The answer will probably be your stuff!

Your wife make you angry? Probably she didn't do something that way YOU wanted. That's your issue!

Your favorite team lose the game? YOU feel depression because YOU chose to take part of your identity from the team's performance. That's your problem!

Your paycheck too small? YOU allowed expenses to grow too big for you to afford. That's YOU!

YOU are 100 percent in charge of how you feel about your life and how it's going! You chose it. And you can choose a different path for your future.

When I finally "heard" Tom, my therapist, I finally understood why he had strapped on steel toed boots at the beginning of every session.

He knew I was too arrogant to acknowledge my responsibility in my life without some serious emotional thrashing from my friends, from him, and especially from my time in depression.

I needed to be smashed down low enough that my dreams could finally look me in the eye and say:

- I messed it up
- I failed to chase them to the end
- I had allowed life to happen to me instead of me happening to my life.

My friend Tony D'Souza calls this *Mindful Living, Choiceful Living.*

When you deal with your stuff, you take huge strides in facing your failures and inevitably learning from them.

As men, one of the most difficult things we have to face is when we've disappointed ourselves. There is no one to blame . . . but ourselves . . . and that sucks.

To learn from our failings is a true test of strength.

If you can learn from your mistakes, improve, and make a better life for yourself, is the failure really that bad?

Face it, most of us men aren't smart enough to figure this stuff out before it's goes bad.

Thus, we have a choice: improve now and do better or repeat our history and screw it all up again . . . Only probably it'll be worse the second time around.

With your life happening now, do you really want to waste it learning a lesson twice?

I spent 14 months in depression. It was a blackness that makes pitch black, child's play. Fortunately, the worst recession since the great depression was going on, because I couldn't get myself to function on most days, so I didn't have to worry about my work suffering.

On the bad days, I was drowning in black tar that encased my soul like the victims from the eruption of Pompeii. On the good days, I was walking blindly through charcoal colored mist. It truly was hell for me.

I can easily imagine that your darkness is hell for you, too.

After walking through all that hell, I can say this:

Depression is a vile force I'd wish on no one . . . and I wouldn't give up my 14 months in it for all the money in the world.

That hell woke me up. It brought a clarity to me and my life that nothing else could.

I now understand my place in the world. I finally feel at home in it.

You can too!

Own your emotional life!

- **RECOGNIZE** your responsibility.
- **RECOGNIZE** your attachments to events, people, places, and/or outcomes.
- **RECOGNIZE** your expectations.

Then, when you acknowledge your stuff, ask yourself **WHY?**

- **WHY** do you have this stuff?
- **WHY** do you expect this outcome?
- **WHY** are you attached to this event, person, place, and/or outcome?

If you need help, seek it and be prepared for steel toed boots. Chances are they will be a harbinger of the best thrashing you could ever allow yourself.

It'll wake you up, force you to live your life, and push you to improve.

If you acknowledge your stuff, own it, and learn from it, you'll start to have the life you wanted.

You'll start to live.

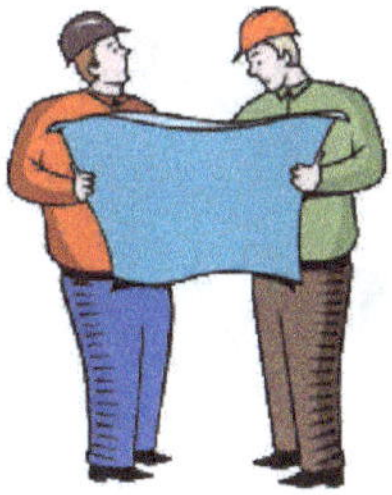

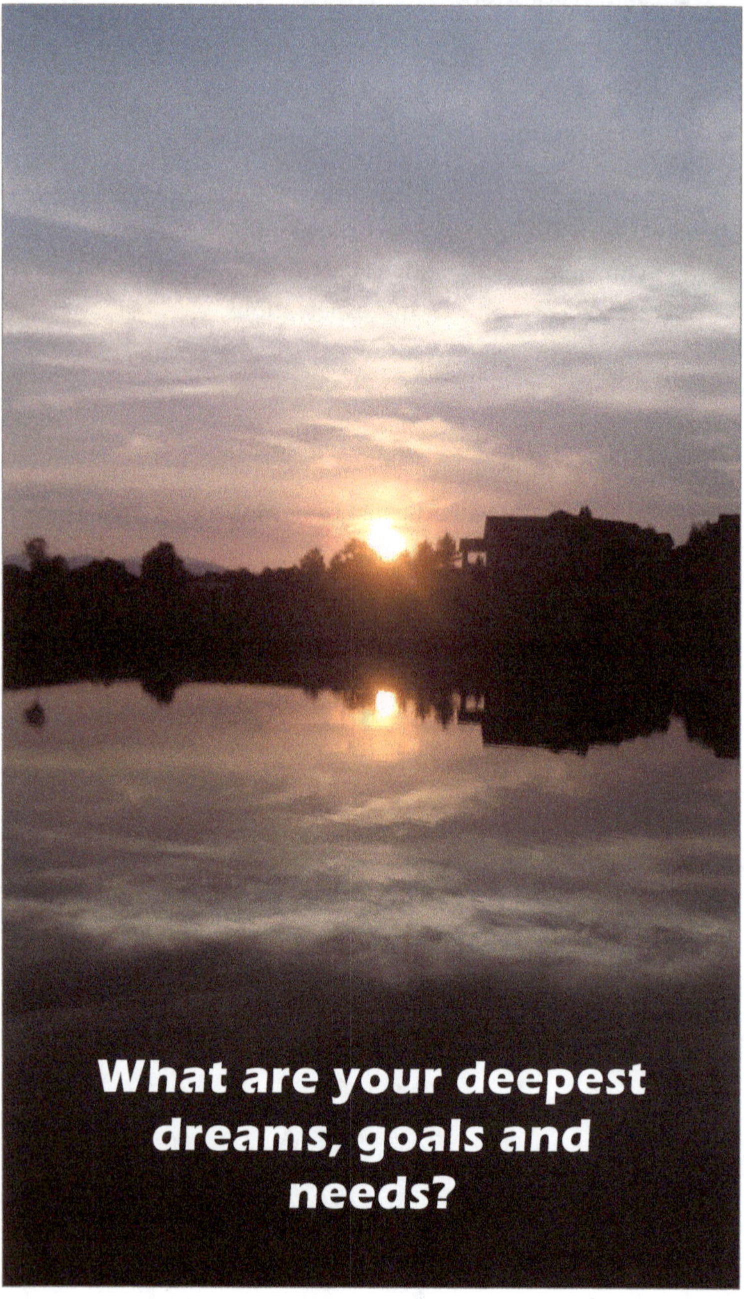

A New Reflection by Blair Ashby

What Do You Really, Really, Really Want

In the summer of 2009, I was sitting in my favorite burrito joint with Tony D'Souza.

I was pissing and moaning about how bad my life was, how unhappy I was, and how much darkness I was living in.

Tony is a very compassionate man. He has a Ph.D. in Psychology and he's a Catholic priest from India who runs a counseling center in Mumbai. He comes to America every year to teach workshops on Awareness and I was fortunate enough to gain him as a client in 1995.

During the past years we've become friends and he is an Awareness mentor to me. This was the first time I'd seen him while I was in depression, though.

He listened to me emotionally bleed for about three hours and then he did something that I completely didn't understand until this year. He picked up a clear cup of water and asked me what I saw. "A cup of water," I said.

He smiled at the idiot I was and asked again what I saw. "A cup of water," I repeated.

He smiled and asked what shape it was.

I now started to think this was some kind of joke. I described the shape of the cup to him and explained that due to water tension and malleability, the water was . . . Ta Da . . . The exact shape of the cup.

I was being a smart ass because I could see nothing but myself when I was in that dark time of my life. Obviously, I knew what shape the water was. I didn't know why he was asking.

Tony then proceeded to make the cleaning personnel work a bit harder. He poured the water out on the floor.

Astounded at the audacity this Indian Priest had, I asked him what the hell he was doing.

He smiled and said, "Blair, what shape is the water?"

I went to get paper napkins to wipe it up. When I returned, I started to bend down to wipe the floor and Tony reached out and stopped me.

"What shape is the water?"

I didn't get it. I asked him to explain his question to me. What was the "deeper" meaning behind the question?

He just smiled for a minute then proceeded to explain something to me which I promptly didn't hear a word of. To this day, I have no idea what he answered me.

I know what I've learned from that episode, though.

A few months before starting this book, I found my

thoughts going back to the water, in the cup and on the floor. You see, I don't know what Tony wanted me to learn, but I know what I've taken from that day. It's like the sound of one hand clapping. You have to define it for yourself. And that is exactly what I learned from the water.

That water was shaped by it's surroundings: the cup, the air when being poured, and then the floor where it came to rest.

Your life is exactly like that water. The difference is, you have a choice on your surroundings. To make decisions on your surroundings, you have to know what kind of boundaries you can live with.

Here is the question in a different way: What do you really, really, really want?

Tony asked that question of me probably fifty times that month he was here in 2009. What do I really, really, really want?

Three really's.

That's extremely important. We aren't talking about boats and cars, or TV's and sports channels. You want those things, but they certainly aren't core to you having a great life. They are fun, yes. But nothing else.

I'm talking about core values here.

- What are your deepest dreams, goals, and needs. Your family, your friends, your career, your legacy?

- Do you have the relationship with your mate you want?
- Do you have the time with your kids that you and they need?
- Do you have a career that fulfills your dreams of a great job?
- Will you be remembered the way you want to be remembered?

And most important, do you have the relationship with yourself you need to thrive?

To say "yes" to any of these, or any other questions that truly reflect your core values, you have to know what you really, really, really want.

In my darkness, I started to take walks. During my blackest days, I'd take three or four walks a day. It was the only thing that helped me get some perspective.

While walking, I'd try and focus my mind on the question of what do I really, really, really want?

At the time, I felt my depression was a direct reflection of being unhappy with my work because I wasn't making any money (never mind the fact it was during the worst economic recession of my lifetime).

So I spent my walks either cursing God for my unhappiness or playing with new career ideas. Sometimes though,

I'd shut up and listen . . .

After yelling at God, the real estate market, Wall Street, the greedy business tycoons, the music industry, the Internet or anything else I could think of to blame for my unhappiness, I'd start to listen to my darkness, my dreams, my goals.

In that listening, I learned I had no idea what I wanted, much less what I really, really, really wanted.

For years, I had lived on the dream of being a big time record producer. The go-to guy (as it were) for the music industry. One day, I had the fortune of meeting and becoming acquaintances with a big time producer.

He talked about what a terrible life he had. Sleeping on a cot in the studio. Not seeing the sun for three weeks on end as they worked 20 hours a day. Flying home Friday night, crashing in bed, and getting up at 4 AM the following Monday to fly out and start it all over again.

All of a sudden, I realized I had no desire to be that person. But I also realized I didn't know what I did want. I had never taken the time to profoundly figure out what I really, really, really wanted. That was a lot of what I thought about when I was walking.

I started out thinking about my career and different careers. I started imagining myself in different careers. Ironically, every career change I imagined came back to mostly what I was doing.

My mind would find a clever way to wrap being an astronaut or fireman back into being a composer/producer/author/speaker who makes all his income from his art.

Eventually, I started to learn I wasn't unhappy with my career. I was unhappy with the amount of money I was making. I was able to finally start seeing myself in the mirror of my reality – in the cup of my life.

I had created boundaries and shapes for myself which I never had any intention of doing. I had made my universe around myself through hundreds of small compromises aiming at a goal that I wasn't even aware of because I had never taken the time to listen to what I really, really, really wanted.

I, then, started to think about what I was thinking about. I started to listen to myself at that point. I learned I valued my alone time in the studio. I valued my creative time, whether it be writing music, or writing essays on my blog. I valued being a confidant to my clients. I valued being thought of as a good listener and a good advice giver. I valued being exactly who I already was but had failed to recognize.

It only took me 43 years to figure this out.

It takes time to understand these things about yourself. Generally, the younger you are, the more time it'll take.

All the previous tools helped me get closer to what I really, really, really wanted.

Let me throw a bit of a wrench into the cogs here.

In my life, and in the lives of the friends whom I talked with about this . . . what we really, really, really want is actually sort of a moving target.

It's not that my aspirations really change so much, as that I grow and open up new possibilities. So what I really, really, really want moves as I learn and experience more.

This book is an example. A year ago, I could never have even dreamed this.

As I got closer to what honestly turned my crank inside, I found, or was introduced to, new ways of chasing my dreams.

A big part of that discovery was actually brought about by the next tool . . .

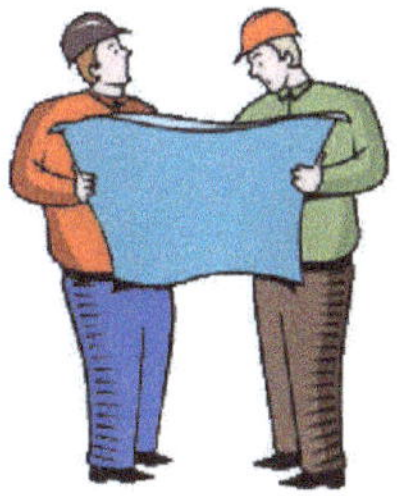

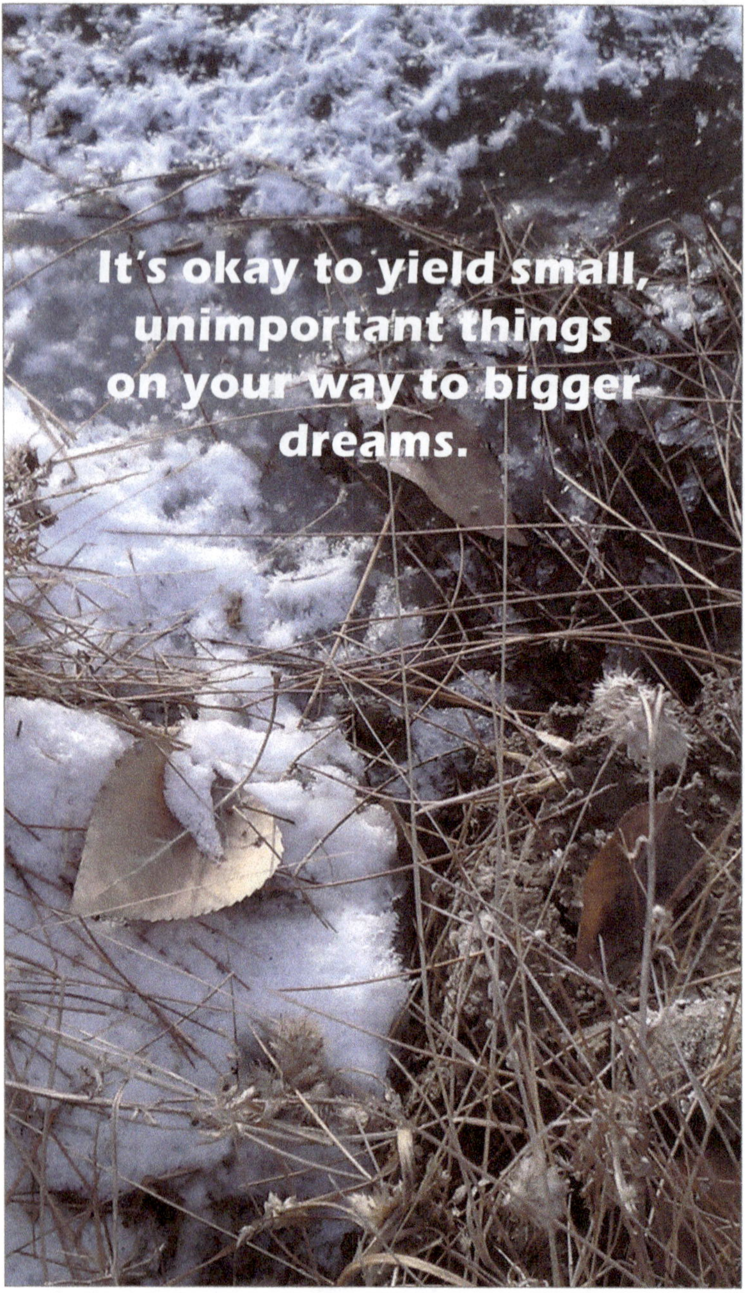
It's okay to yield small,
unimportant things
on your way to bigger
dreams.

Snow, Weed, Ice, Leaf by Blair Ashby

Winning By Yielding

"What do you really, really, really want?" is probably the most important thing I've ever learned in my life. It shapes everything I now do.

Every decision I make, every career move I make, every weekend activity I get involved in all comes back to: What do you really, really, really want, Blair?

This, however, meant nothing to me until two years after Tony asked me that question. I needed to hear another story before I could fully grasp the true meaning of "What do I really, really, really want?"

Scott has been a friend of mine since I was seven years old. At times, he's been a good friend and other times, he's been one of the best friends I've ever had.

One afternoon in 2011, after a great pizza lunch, he told me about driving home from work everyday.

He described his route and the corner at which he turns north onto a two lane road that, 150 feet later, collapses into one lane. He told me how turning drivers race as fast as they can to try and get one car ahead in the long line of cars going up the hill on that one lane road. He told me about how he used to do that and how many times he felt like he was taking a chance by squeezing his truck into an opening fit for only a small car. He went on to say that, then, one day he had a light bulb go on.

What he wanted was to get home and see his wife and kids. He could only do this if he was safe.

If he just waited until the cross-traffic light changed, he could turn directly into the continuous lane with no risk to his life or truck. He could then drive home less stressed and arrive safely to his waiting wife and family in a much better mood.

He realized that he was missing the bigger goal to accomplish a small one! He called this: Winning by Yielding. I call this brilliant!

But, winning by yielding only works if you know what you really, really, really want.

Remember the hundreds of little sacrifices you made to get where you are now?

Maybe you sacrificed seeing a few games of your kids so you could get "ahead" at a past job from which you can't even remember your boss' name. Now your kids are grown and there are no games of theirs to see. Was it worth it?

Darkness comes from thinking like that...

Now look at this a different way. You are spending a lot of time and effort learning about yourself and what you really, really, really want.

In the future, keep your dreams first and foremost and wrap your decisions around them. Instead of letting life happen to you, you happen to life.

Once Scott knew he wanted to arrive home safe and in a good mood to see his wife and kids, he could easily sacrifice being one car ahead.

The fact is, if you know your bigger goals you can compromise the smaller goals without sacrificing your dreams.

It's sometimes called losing a battle to win a war.

And for me, "What do I really, really, really want?" meant nothing until I learned "Winning by yielding."

That was when I finally understood what Tony was doing with the water.

Life is full of compromise and sacrifice. It cannot be helped. Many times, life forces itself on us.

However, if we are cognizant of what our bigger goals and dreams are, we can shape our decisions and boundaries to better fit our needs.

Tony calls it *Mindful Living, Choiceful Living.*

Scott calls it *Winning by Yielding.*

The military calls it *Losing a battle to win a war.*

I don't care what name you give it.

It's making good decisions based on knowing what your ultimate goal is.

It's taking control of your life with a healthy respect for the reality of compromise in life.

And no matter what you call it, it's good living.

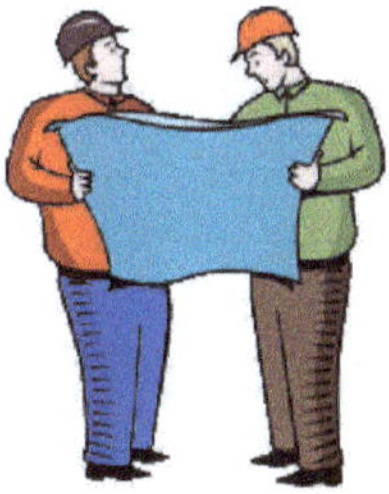

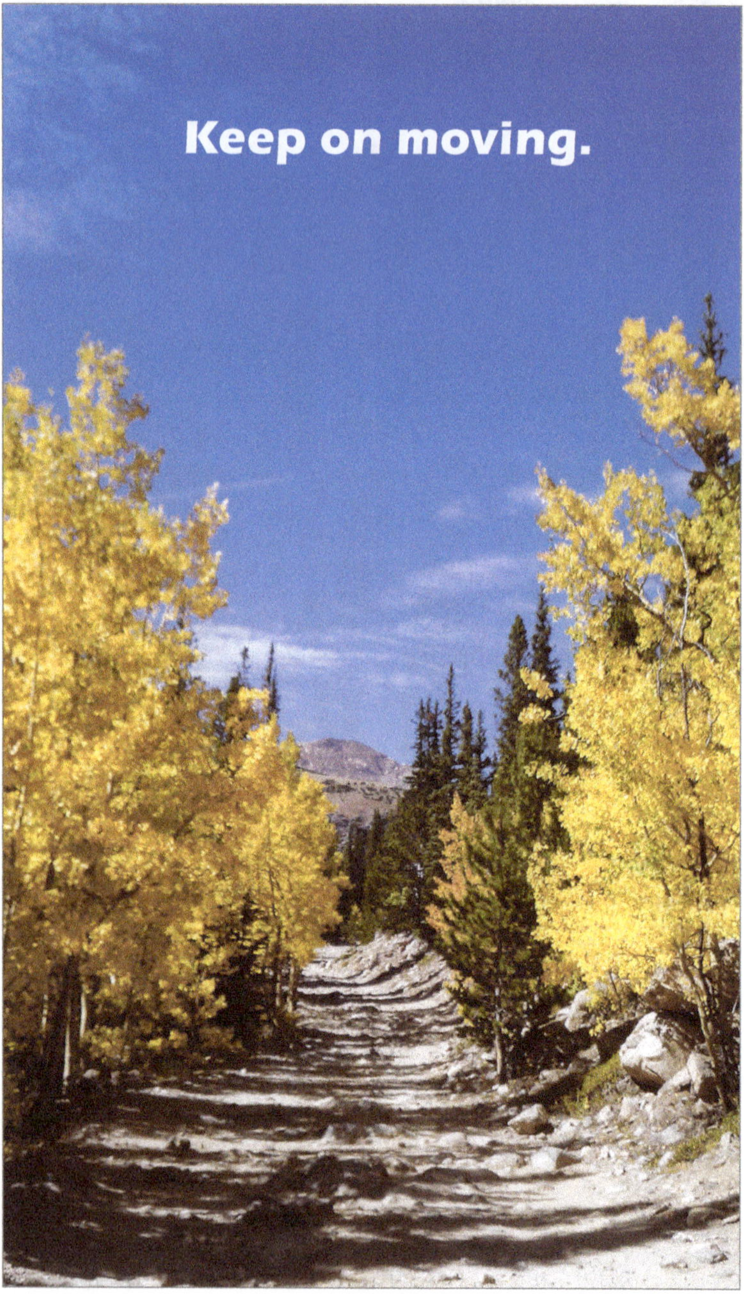

St. Mary's Alice by Blair Ashby

Keep Looking In The Mirror

Hopefully . . .

You've put your fingers on the wall and started to move.

If you haven't yet, hopefully you will, and let yourself feel the burn, the darkness, the anger, and the loneliness.

It will suck, but you will learn from it!

You are not your emotions, you only feel them.

If you shut up, you will give your dreams a chance to speak to you.

From all this quiet misery, you should start to get a better sense of your life.

You'll, hopefully, start to get some semblance of control back in your reality.

You'll start to get epiphanies on what you really, really, really want and how to get there.

You'll see the small unimportant goals you can sacrifice to reach the big dreams in your life.

It all takes time, but if you deal with your own stuff, force yourself to look at you with a powerful microscope, and start fixing your life, you will have a great future!

When you reach the point of rebuilding your life the way you want – chasing your dreams, going for and accomplishing your goals – it's extremely important to learn from your past.

Now, more than ever, you need to keep looking in the mirror. You have to constantly ask yourself two questions:

- "What is my stuff (in this situation)?" and
- "What do I really, really, really want?"

If you don't learn from your history, you will repeat it…and it will suck even more out of you the next time.

If you remember, in describing the previous tools, I talked about what you want being sort of a like a moving target.

Chances are, your actual dreams will stay the same, but your methods of living those dreams will expand as you get to know your life and the Universe better.

In my life, I started out aiming in the right direction towards being creative, but then got distracted by the glory and perceived rewards of being a big time music producer.

In fact, I wanted to be valued for my knowledge and experience, not my image as a go-to music man.

Because I had failed to examine my motives by asking myself why I did anything, I became entranced by the perceived notion of being valued as the 'save the band' music producer.

If I had focused some good, quiet time on my motivations early in my career, I might have learned my true dreams and stayed better focused on them. I might even have avoided the 14 months of depression and 16 months of therapy I went through.

Instead, I drifted off into the world of image and false goals for my life. I have met producers who were born to be big time producers. They are living their dreams to the fullest. I do not want to be one of them. Yet, as I failed to examine myself, I tried to make myself a part of their world.

I thank my lucky star I had my depression and darkness. It forced me to look at myself and find my true motivations. It forced me to ask myself why.

From that beginning, I could navigate the darkness of depression and push through to the life on the other side.

Now, I owe it to myself to always look in the personal mirror of my soul to ask myself, "What is my stuff? Why am I doing this or that? What is my ultimate goal?" To search out my motivations and deal with them whether good or bad.

Then I ask myself, "What do I really, really, really want? By reacting to this situation, will I further my own personal goals or am I reacting to a perceived threat to my image or security? Instead, if I respond proactively to the situation, can I create a win/win scenario that furthers everyone's goals, including mine?"

By constantly looking in the mirror of my own reality, I can weigh in on my motivations and goals. I can judge if I'm enriching my life or only furthering my ego. I can have my eyes wide open. I can choose to thrive, not just survive.

You must be willing to examine yourself relentlessly under the powerful microscope of your dreams or core values.

Your core values are like a GPS in your soul.

If you watch them, you can constantly make the fine adjustments needed to keep yourself on the path you choose to be on. If you forget about them, the day will come when they lead you back into darkness to try and get your attention.

Quiet times in your own world spent looking at yourself are invaluable.

- Go play some ball in the driveway,
- Work on the car.
- Mow the lawn.
- Hike a mountain.

Do anything that gives you some time to "Shut up and

listen to yourself!" It will be rewarding beyond measure.

Taking some time each day to ask yourself "Why?" will let you create the life that you want to live.

Dedicating an hour each week to asking, "What do I really, really, really want?" will allow you to focus your mind on each situation in your life and make conscious decisions about your role in them.

You will have more control in your life as you respond pro-actively to your life instead of responding reactively to life.

Take the time so you can live.

Constantly allow your inner GPS to function so you can stay true to your goals, your dreams, your core values, your life.

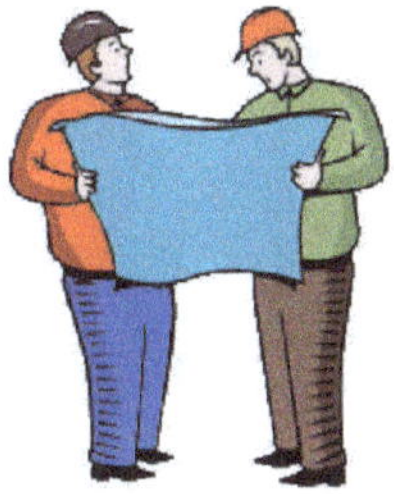

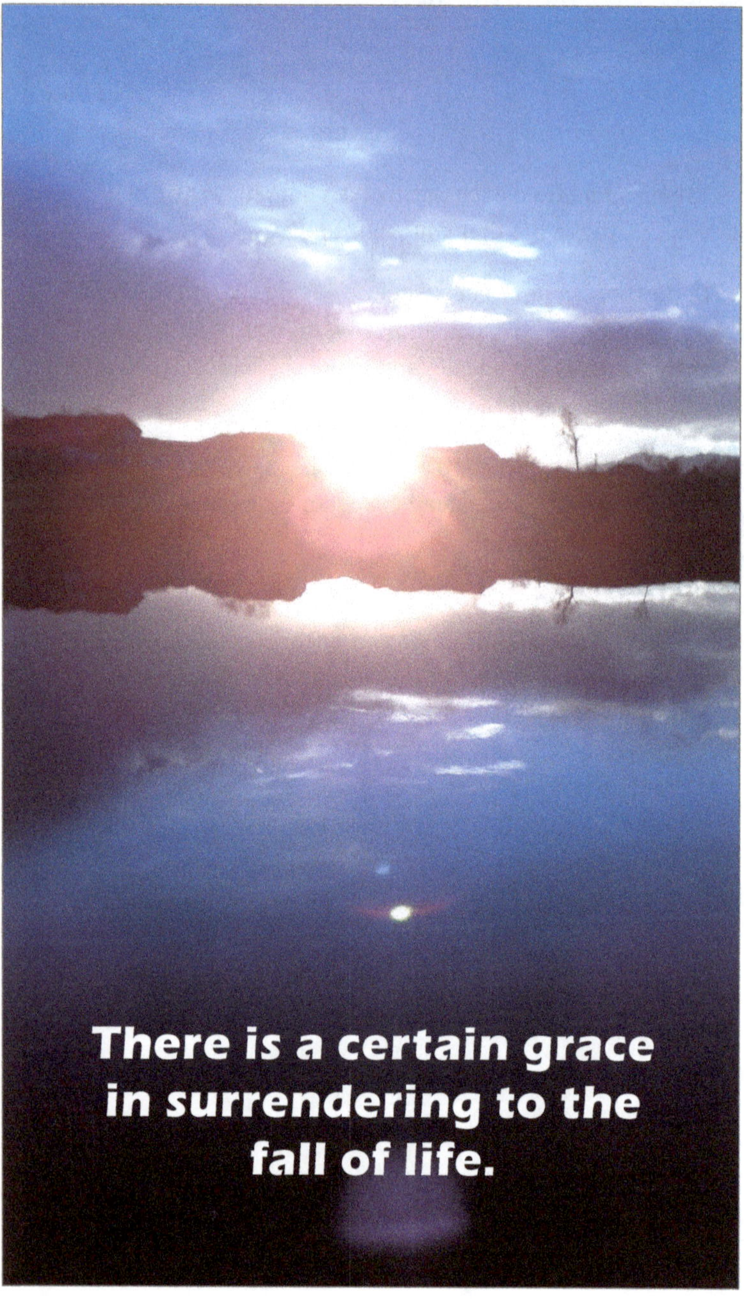

Bright Sunrise by Blair Ashby

Never Stop Falling

In January of 2012, I recorded Rabbi Shapiro speaking to a room full of Christians about the contemplative nature of spirituality.

I am not a religious person at all. I am, however, a pretty spiritual person, and I've had the honor to record many of the worlds greatest spiritual minds over the past twenty years.

I've recorded Rabbi Shapiro before and I've found him to be a particularly deep thinker. I like how he challenges me to go beyond my preconceived notions of reality and spirituality.

In this specific conference, he was talking about the ancient nature of God, the Universe, or whatever label you want to give it.

The pivotal point for me was when he looked out on the large audience and said, " . . . You Christians have got it all wrong. You always talk about the arms of God supporting you when you trip. You talk about one set of footprints in the sand when God carries you. You say God will catch you when you fall off a cliff. You seem to think that God is waiting at the bottom with his arms wide open, ready for you to gently land in them! . . ."

He went on to rock my world with his next statement: " . . . People, God is not at the bottom. God is not going to carry you. God is not going to catch you. God is the fall! He is always catching you! God is! Period!"

Please understand, I don't want to go all spiritual on you. I haven't up to this point and I won't start now. Let me, instead, frame Rabbi Shapiro's statement in a non-spiritual light.

As men, we frequently feel out of place in the world.

We are only recently down from the trees, as Thomas Keating says. We aren't equipped to handle the modern world we men have created.

I often have men tell me how lost they feel. Caught up in our bosses' demands, the honey-do list, the 'you should be here at this time,' the lawsuits, the cool cars, the down from the home team losing, and all the obligations – we feel deflated and powerless to control our destiny.

Men, life is a constant fall. We are never fully in control of our lives.

The minute we can walk, we are told, "don't go there" or "do come here." We grow up with people always telling us how to behave, how to not behave, where to go and when, what to wear, what not to wear, the beer to drink, and the food real men don't eat.

We are battered left and right by forces that frequently we can't even see.

Life is a constant fall. Keep falling! It's okay.

The purpose of this book is to give you some tools to help you trust yourself in that fall.

Life is always catching you. You will not hit the ground and break into a million pieces, nor will you splat out like a bug on the windshield.

If you stay aware of your goals, your dreams, your core values, you have a say in how you fall.

Some things we can never control. We can accept that. Fall, and trust it'll be okay. We can, though, know ourselves and trust ourselves to choose the direction we fall in, as much as possible.

We are all made exactly as the universe wanted us. Whether we call it a fortuitous accident of evolution or a divine creation, we are exactly as we should be.

Do you think for one minute that the universe made you the way it doesn't want you to be?

What do you really, really, really, want? If you follow that dream, you will be and do exactly what you're supposed to be and do.

Amazingly, when we follow that dream, we find our place in the universe, in our relationships, in our careers, with our friends, in our lives.

When we accept our dreams as the way we should be, we come home in the fall that is life. We find rest in the fall. We find peace in the constant change, knowing it'll be okay. We trust the forces beyond our control to work out in a way best for us.

I like to say God draws straight with crooked lines.

Maybe a better way to say it is, life draws straight with crooked lines.

If we are able to accept life as it comes, we give life more room to draw straight, which almost always benefits us.

Conversely, the more we try to micro-control our reality, the more we fight life and fail. There is no way we can know all the dynamic variables involved in all the threads that create our reality. There are just too many people we interact with, too many motivations, too many thoughts, and too many other realities.

There is a certain grace in surrendering to the fall of life. You stop fighting to control every nuance. You stop wasting energy on trying to change unchangeable things.

My friend, Warren, says fighting to control the uncontrollable is heat and light. It's wasted energy.

I suspect you have watched people you know try to influence situations or people and all that happened was exactly what the controller didn't want to happen.

If this wasn't a faulty part of humanity, we wouldn't have so many television shows about it to distract us from our own lives. TV stories are built on our desire to control everything.

Life is a fall.

One long, amazing fall.

Of course, this is said by a man who went through a horrible darkness and learned to accept, surrender, trust, welcome, and feel grateful and humble for that very darkness.

It gave me the fortitude to move through the exact things that were killing me. It, then, gave me the tools to rebuild my life in a way more congruent with my goals, dreams, and core values.

The Minnesota folk singer, Peter Mayer, wrote a song called *God is a River*. In it he describes the human desire to cling to a rock against the onslaught of the mighty river.

Eventually, though, we learn the rock is not a salvation but rather a hindrance to living in the flow of the river.

Instead, let go. Watch all the amazing scenery and experiences that go with being in the flow. Why would we think we'd have a better life clutching an immovable rock, battered by the constant rush of the flow dragging at our bodies?

If you go with the flow, you feel very little pressure from the water, and yet, because you can swim, you can control the direction you travel in.

Keep falling. Your dreams are always catching you. You will not die from the darkness you have to walk through to get to your life.

Instead . . . maybe . . .

Just maybe . . .

Your dreams pushed you off the cliff of your old life into the darkness just so they could catch you.

All the way down to a better life.

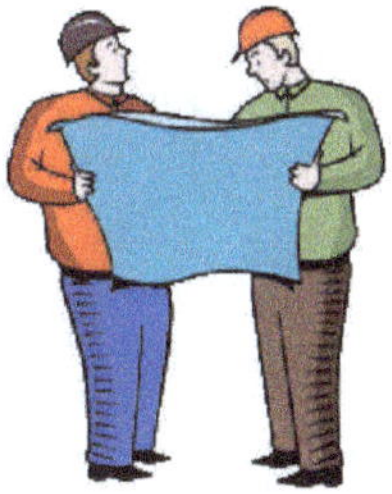

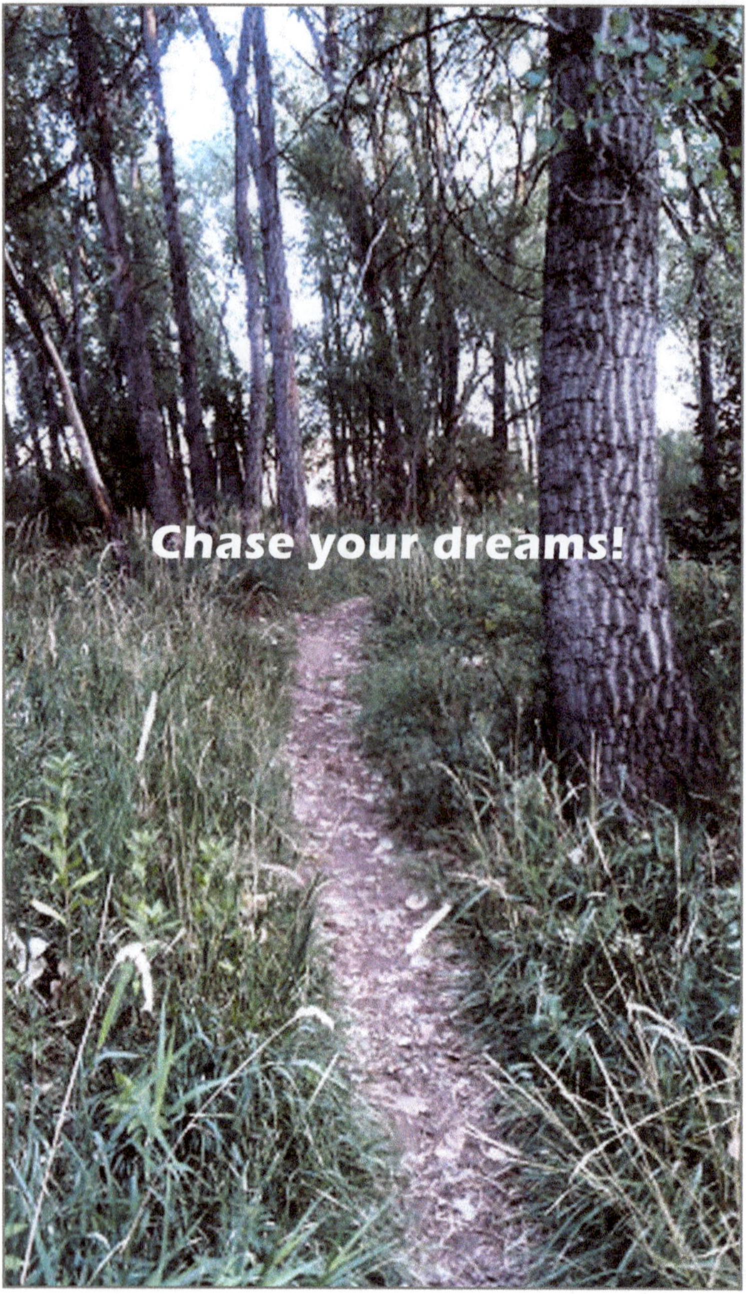

Rock Creek Path by Blair Ashby

Afterword

by Jim Rae, Ph.D.

"Men" . . . We have a tendency to want to solve all of our problems in the private confines of our minds. It is not unusual for us to wait until we are deep in the bowels of our own discontent before we begin to search for the reasons why. Asking for help and guidance is not an easy thing for us to do, particularly when we are running on empty.

We can be very skilled at justifying our actions or inactions with regards to our unique personal pain and suffering. This is especially true when we find ourselves in those desperate situations where there are no answers, no viable solutions, and nothing seems to matter.

Seeking help in our darkest hours is as foreign for us, at times, as it is for us to share our deepest, most intimate feelings with another. It seems as if we are genetically hard-wired to solve our personal problems completely by ourselves. We are problem solvers, damnit! God forbid we find ourselves in a lonely, dark place feeling depressed and totally helpless.

One of my professors in graduate school, Dr. Jon Winterton, spent five years researching "luck." He examined luck to see if he could identify any connection between good luck and happiness, and bad luck and sadness. Dr. Winterton's research concluded with the following: "*Good things happen to those who are in motion!*"

Action, any kind of action, is better than no action, especially when we believe we have hit a critical roadblock or dead end. If we remain motionless, we will drastically decrease our chances and opportunities to discover new possibilities. By taking extremely small steps, we will slowly begin to see our reality from a different perspective.

As Blair has so clearly stated in *Talking Man to Man*, there are no quick fixes, or immediate cures for deep darkness. When everything you have tried has failed and you find yourself emotionally drained, muster the courage to ask for help and pay attention to your internal compass, the one deep inside of you, that is always right, but not always followed.

Listen for your *true north* and take that first small step and then another . . . Go after what you "really, really, really want."

Chase Your Dreams!

Acknowledgements

It's impossible to name all the people and dynamic variables that helped bring this book to fruition.

I wrote this book in 2012 to the *me I was in 2009* when I fell into depression. However, the information in this book was learned from all the amazing gifts of time and words that countless sages have given to me over the past twenty years and especially during the past five years.

My friend, Tony D'Souza was invaluable, especially his book and video series *Discovering Awareness*. Tony spent thirty days with me in the summer of 2009 which still echo in my life. "What do you really, really, really want?" is his gift. Thank you, Tony.

Jim Rae called me in 2009 and offered me a job opportunity which changed my way of thinking. I didn't take the job, but I didn't forget it either. It looks like you were probably four years early Jim!

Nancy Smith at *Sounds True* gave me the first inkling that a book existed in me and her idea planted the seed which grew into the book you're now reading.

Robert Korotky took me to the conference which taught

me my gift with words and my weakness at back office production. Yes, Rob, that was money well spent! Because, when Fred Berns walked into my studio a week later and told me I needed to write and talk about my experience, I was ready to hear it, knowing I needed other people and their back office strengths to help me.

Fred, I can't say thank you enough! You were the final catalyst who brought all the ideas together and formed them into a manageable plan. You gave my ideas direction while focusing me on the need for delivering this message.

Terri Murphy used gallons of red ink making this readable. She compassionately made suggestions for improvement which every reader will appreciate, even though they might not realize it. You are a gift to writers everywhere and especially to this wordsmith.

E&R Publishing took Fred's idea and made it tangible and colorful. The formatting came about through weeks of tossing ideas back and forth with my editor until I felt like this was the book I wish I had had in my darkness.

Finally, my mom and dad made sure I ate in the final three weeks of writing. Thanks so much, Mom, for your support during the last five years and the writing of this book.

Thank you all for the amazing gifts you all have given me.

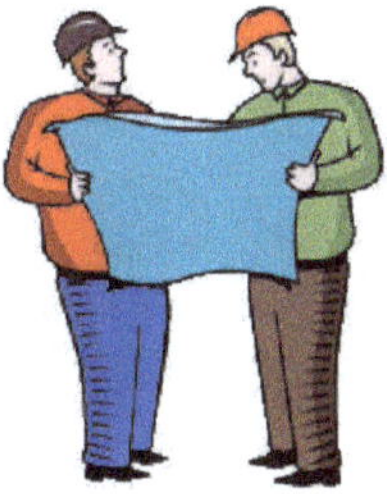

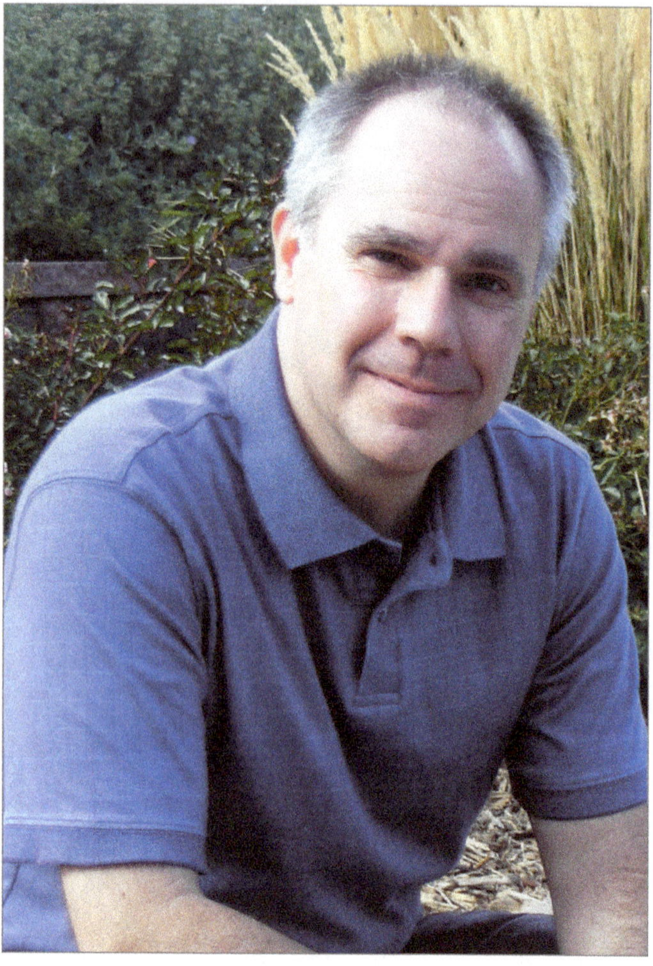

Photograph by Kira Groves

About The Author

Blair Ashby is an audio and music producer, author, and general "go with the flow" kind of guy. He has a communication degree and is only two lab classes short of his psychology degree. However, after 14 months of depression and 16 months of therapy, he's fairly certain that he's smarter than the mice he would have studied and he's more than qualified for the degree now, anyway.

When he's not lecturing, writing books, blogging, or composing music, you can generally find him recording many of the finest spiritual thinkers who come to Denver.

Read Blair's blog at www.BlairAshby.com
or email him at TMTM@BlairAshby.com

CPSIA information can be obtained
at www.ICGtesting.com
Printed in the USA
LVHW06s1259170418
573799LV00013B/241/P

9 780984 737376